CHINESE HERBAL MEDICINE FOR BEGINNERS

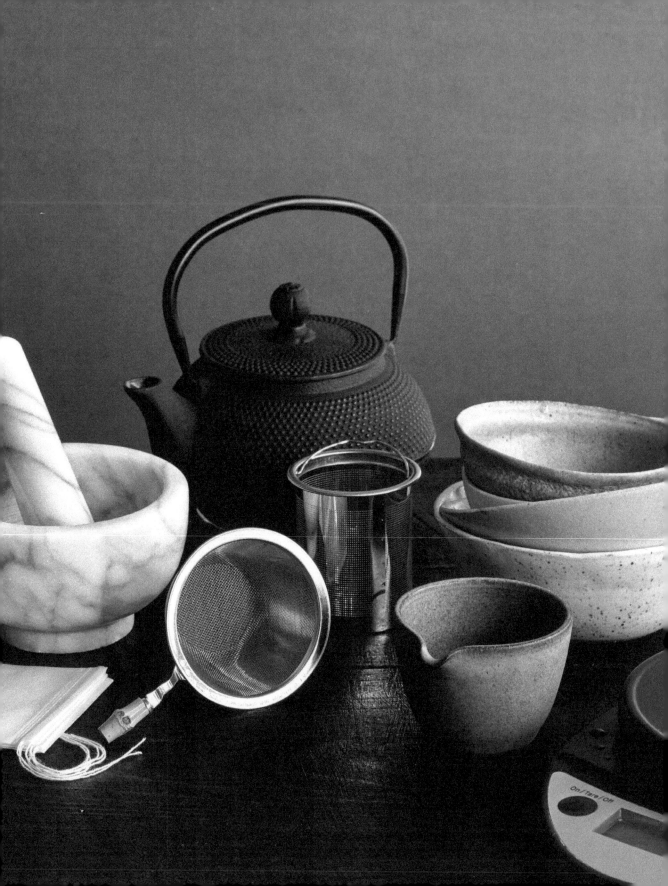

Chinese Herbal Medicine

for BEGINNERS

Over 100 Remedies for Wellness and Balance

Carrie Chauhan

Photography by Biz Jones

ROCKRIDGE
PRESS

Interior and Cover Designer: Julie Gueraseva
Art Producer: Michael Hardgrove
Editor: Samantha Barbaro
Production Editor: Mia Moran
Custom Photography © 2020 Biz Jones
Food styling by Erika Joyce
Interior art used under license from © Shutterstock.com & iStockphoto.com
Author photo courtesy of © Wendy Wood Photography

ISBN: Print 978-1-64611-413-9 | eBook 978-1-64611-414-6
R0

With love to Anuj and Akshay

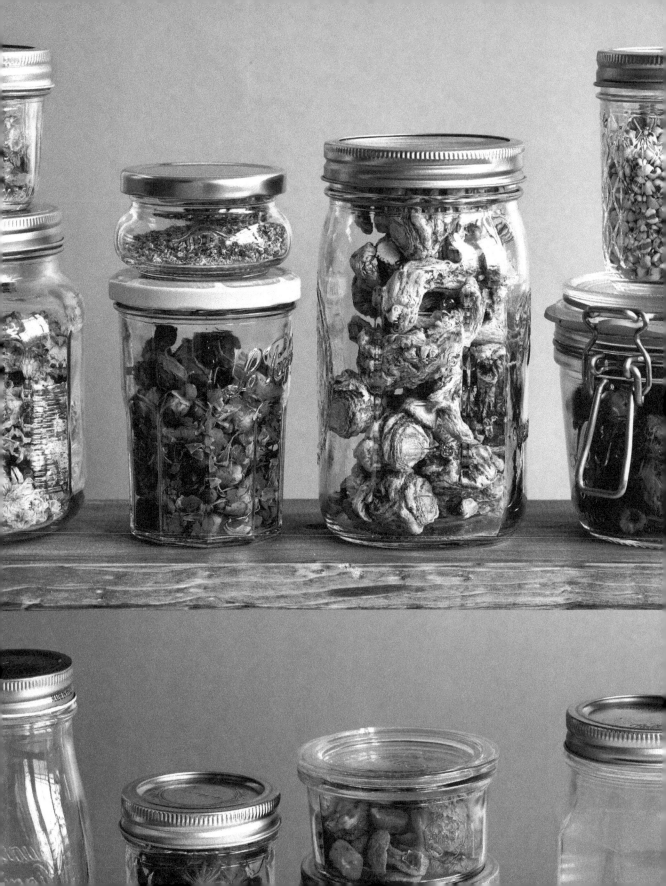

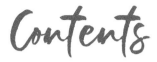

Contents

PART III: Formulas and Remedies 67

CHAPTER 4: FORMULAS AND REMEDIES 69

Introduction

I love herbal medicine, no matter the system or where it originated. Plants are amazing. I started reading about and experimenting with herbal medicine on my own, using books much like this one. Before becoming a practitioner of Chinese medicine, I taught yoga therapy and Ayurveda. While completing my degree in acupuncture and Chinese herbal medicine, I worked at a GNC store, helping people with herbs and supplements. I also volunteered my limited free time to help my teachers and supervisors by working in the herbal dispensary making formulas for patients. I just wanted to be in the dispensary, a room filled with more than 300 jars of herbs, each with a different smell, look, and feel. When I opened the door, the aroma of all those herbs mixed together would draw me in. During school, my acupuncture performance was fine, but everyone knew my true love lay in Chinese herbal medicine.

After graduation, I continued to learn more about herbal medicine by enrolling in an Ayurvedic course, and I also joined the American Herbalist Guild to learn Western herbal medicine. At the same time, I was beginning my Chinese medicine practice and working at the Academy for Five Element Acupuncture as dispensary manager, herb clinic supervisor, teacher, and eventually director. My passion is working directly with students and herbs.

Even though I know other systems of herbal medicine, 99 percent of the time I use the Chinese system to diagnose, because I find it so thorough and exacting in getting to the root of any problem. Currently, I'm working with a colleague using locally grown Western herbs according to the principles of Chinese medicine. I'm excited about the future of Chinese herbal medicine in the United States.

Western herbalist Rosemary Gladstar summed up herbalists and herbalism in general when she said, "The only thing herbalists can agree on is not to cook your herbs in an aluminum pan." Herbal medicine comes from all over the world, forged in different cultures and used in a variety of ways. Herbal medicine has made some pretty big things happen in my life, and I've seen it do amazing things for my clients, family, and friends. I hope this book helps you explore and find what works best for you.

My goal in writing this book is to make the vastness of Chinese medicine digestible for a beginner and to make its systems of diagnosis approachable. You will get a sense of how you can use Chinese herbal medicine to decide which herb to use and when, and how it will help you fortify your health and thrive!

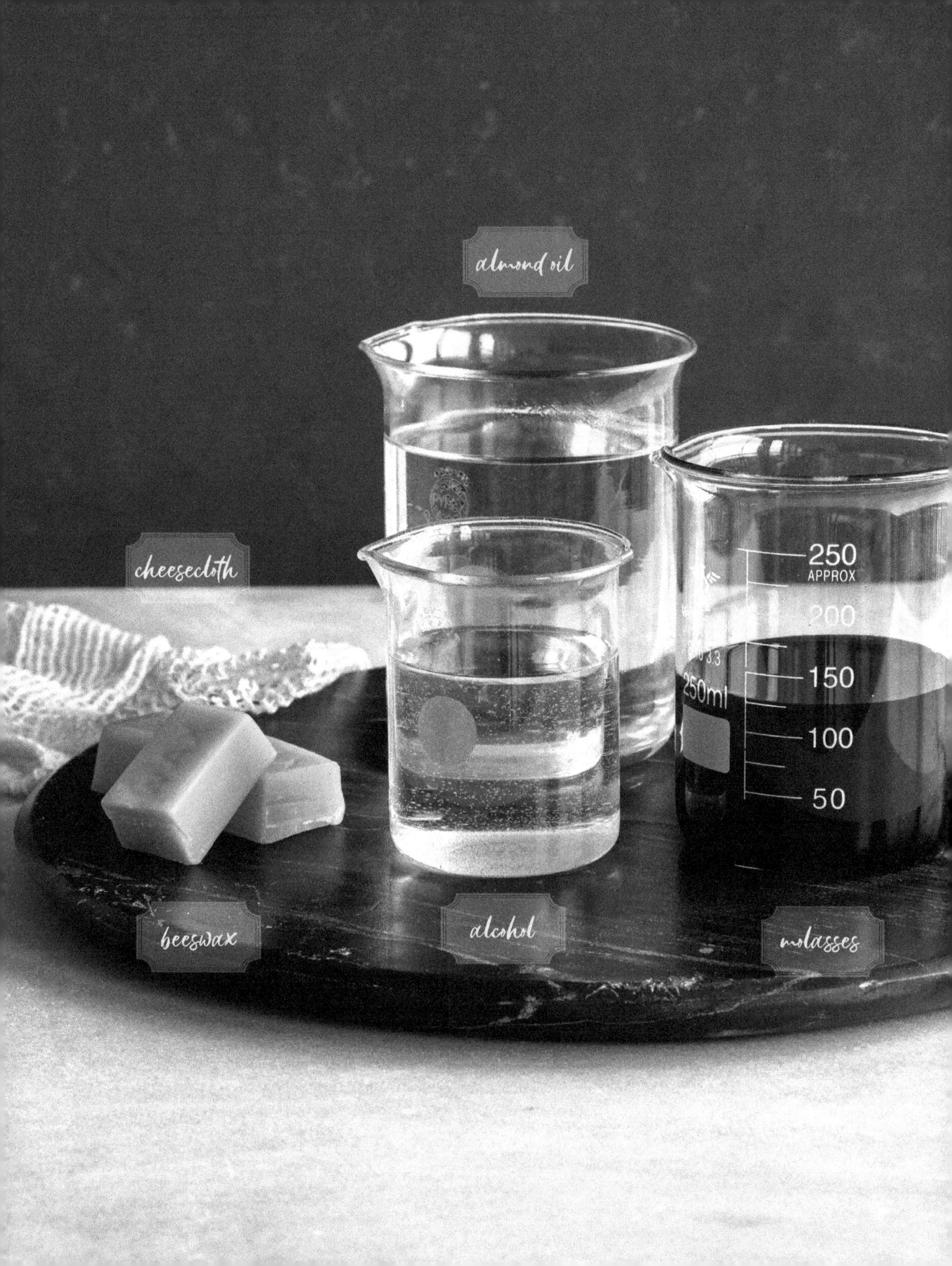

almond oil

cheesecloth

beeswax

alcohol

250
APPROX

200

150

100

50

0.3

250ml

molasses

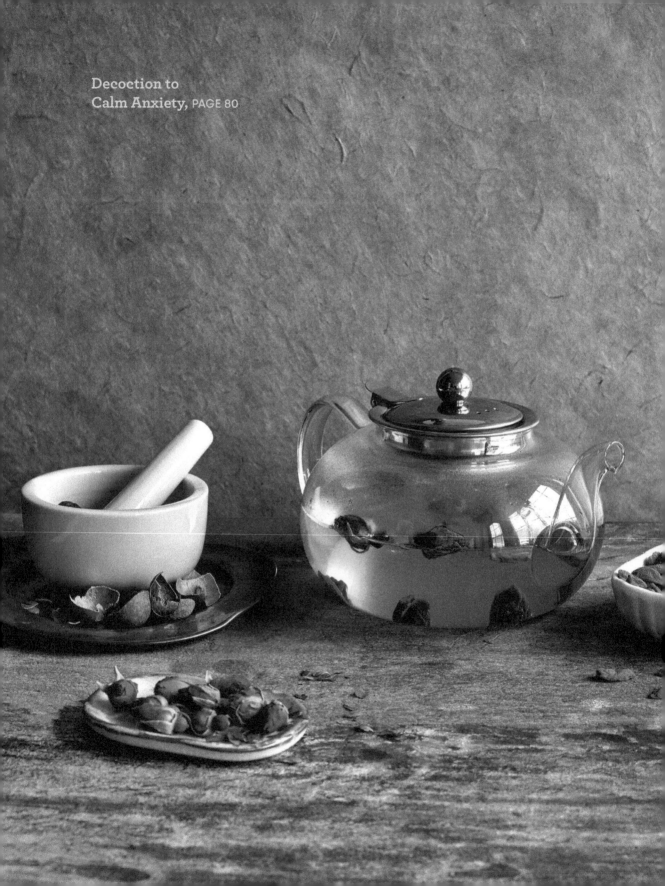

Decoction to
Calm Anxiety, PAGE 80

Part One

YOUR CHINESE HERBAL MEDICINE PRIMER

Because it is a system of holistic healing, Chinese herbal medicine does not seek to cure Western medical diagnoses. Rather, its main focus is preventing illness by maintaining balance physically, mentally, and spiritually. It helps disease and illness by the same mechanism of restoring balance, being therapeutically gentle or strong depending on what is needed.

This book is designed to break down the vastness that is Chinese herbal medicine into simple first steps toward learning the system. The first chapter introduces you to the basic concepts of Chinese herbal medicine. At first, the Chinese medical framework may seem daunting to learn, but looking at health and disease through this lens allows for thorough, detailed understanding of many conditions. This depth of understanding allows for an equally exacting plan of treatment for the condition patterns. In chapter 2, you will explore setting up your home apothecary, which will include the Chinese herbs from chapter 3 to make the formulas or remedies in chapter 4.

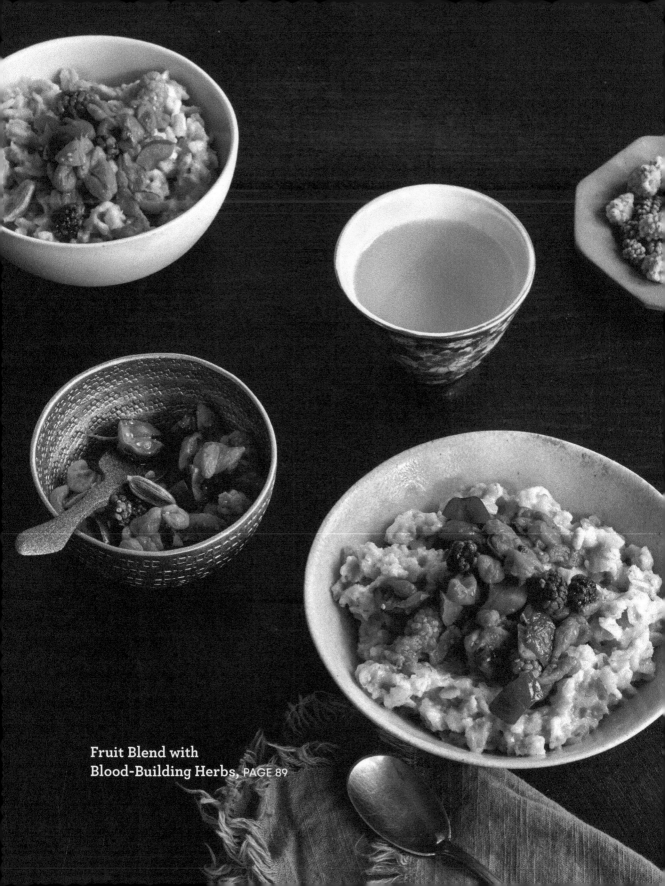

Fruit Blend with
Blood-Building Herbs, PAGE 89

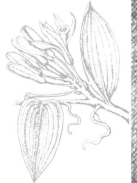

CHAPTER 1

All about Chinese Herbal Medicine

Before we get into the herbs and remedies, there are some important concepts to cover first. These concepts work together to form the Chinese system of differentiation and diagnosis that sets Chinese herbal medicine apart. The ability to thoroughly distinguish between all of the various underlying causes of a condition, accurately diagnose, and prescribe elegant and precise herbal formulas is the wonder that is Chinese herbal medicine. In this chapter, you will learn the foundational elements of Chinese medicine so you can confidently move forward to creating your apothecary and making formulas.

What Is Chinese Herbal Medicine?

Chinese herbal medicine is a traditional system of healing from Asia dating back thousands of years. It is the branch of Traditional Chinese Medicine that uses plants in the form of roots, berries, leaves, and barks to treat imbalances and disease. Perfected over centuries, these medicinals are mixed together and used in combinations called formulas that can contain up to 18 ingredients.

Traditional systems of medicine have no known start dates. Some of the earliest records are from the Han Dynasty in China, which lasted from AD 25 to 220. These writings recorded what already existed at the time, which means the system dates back even further. Chinese herbal medicine was already a working system of medicine that continued to develop. During the later Tang Dynasty, a surviving *Materia Medica* collected information on almost 850 herbs in use. A *Materia Medica* is a book that lists herbal medicines, their medicinal uses, and other information. Throughout this long history of use, Chinese herbal medicine has continued to grow and develop, but when learning this medicine, students still read classics like Huang Di's *Nei Jing Su Wen*.

Chinese herbal medicine gives you the tools to work toward balance and to keep your body, mind, and spirit healthy. It helps you be the best version of yourself. Chinese medicine uses nature as the ideal of balance in multiple systems that are intertwined. My favorite metaphor of how holistic healing works compares people to trees. In health, not everyone will be a robust oak tree. Some are short, round apple trees, while others are tall, thin pine trees. The beauty of holistic systems of healing is that our health goals are unique to us individually, and we are not held to standards that are impossible to attain.

As you learn the basic theory of Chinese herbal medicine, keep in mind that it is a framework through which you can see the whole world—and yourself and others. Remember that this is an introduction to the principles: You could study this medicine your entire life and never find the end point where you declare, "Yes, I know it all." With deep, ancient history comes a lot of information. But despite centuries of different writers and teachers and scholars, the basics remain the same. They are simple but can be applied to almost anything.

Traditional Chinese Medicine

TCM stands for Traditional Chinese Medicine. Today in the United States, TCM is often used as a general term referring to Chinese medicine. While we talk about China as its country of origin, throughout history other countries such as Korea and Japan found this medicine (or it migrated to them). Centuries ago, they took Chinese medicine and made it their own, so it can also be referred to as *Asian Medicine*. I find this to be a more accurate term, as Asian countries such as Japan and Korea have made valuable contributions to the field.

Traditional Chinese Medicine includes Chinese herbal medicine, acupuncture, cupping, tui na, gua sha, nutrition, and moxibustion.

Acupuncture is the insertion of extremely thin needles—thinner than a human hair—into specific points on the body. These points are located on one of the 12 energetic pathways known as meridians. These points affect the flow of energy through the meridians and can help relieve symptoms while promoting health and balance. A way of imagining meridians is as a subway map to a large city like London or Berlin. There are multiple lines that can take you all over, with designated stops and places where lines meet or cross. The acupuncture meridians travel through the body this way, reaching the extremities and providing hundreds of points where the energy of the meridians can be accessed.

Most practitioners use multiple therapies in a single appointment: You might receive moxibustion, acupuncture, and another therapy like cupping or tui na as well as an herbal formula to take home with you. Moxibustion (or "moxa") uses the dried herb mugwort (*Artemisia vulgaris*), which is formed into cones and warmed to stimulate acupuncture points. Moxibustion excels at reducing inflammation, increasing energy, and relieving pain. Tui na, gua sha, and cupping are hands-on treatments. Tui na is a massage that balances and clears the acupuncture meridians, while gua sha releases tension, stagnation, and heat. Cupping, which involves applying suction to a meridian, acupuncture point, or muscular area, has become more well known since famous Olympians appeared onscreen with the unmistakably perfect circular red marks.

CHINESE HERBAL MEDICINE TODAY

Today's Chinese herbal medicine is varied. Some practitioners are more traditional: They are dedicated to helping patients stay healthy or treat diseases and disharmonies exclusively using TCM.

Chinese herbal medicine can also look more modern, with Chinese herbal practitioners integrated within Western medical settings such as clinics, hospitals, chiropractic offices, and cancer treatment programs. The Cleveland Clinic even has a Chinese herbal medicine program.

LEARNING THE BASICS

Chinese herbal medicine is learned as part of a four-year master's degree program in Traditional Chinese Medicine and is learned alongside acupuncture, tui na, moxibustion, and other modalities. To practice Chinese medicine in the United States, at minimum you need a master's degree, but doctoral programs are developing and becoming more widely available. Once you have your degree, you then pass multiple exams to become nationally certified and then certified in the state where you practice.

Modern practitioners are also more inclined to specialize, focusing on areas like fertility and reproductive health or cancer treatment. Along with these specializations can come an extra level of certification, like being certified by ABORM, the American Board of Oriental Reproductive Medicine, for fertility specialists.

Whether someone has a specialty or general practice, a master's or a doctorate, the education is based on the same concepts and systems developed through the centuries.

ANIMAL PARTS

You may have read about animal parts in Chinese herbal medicine. While this book does not advocate the use of animal parts, historically, Chinese herbal medicine used animal products, including some from exotic species like the rhinoceros. It's easy to understand why sourcing these products without endangering animal populations would be a challenge. Where animal parts have historically been used, plenty of plants can be used in their place.

The Principles of Chinese Herbal Medicine

Herbalism has more depth than simple memes on social media that tell you a certain herb is for a certain condition. As we explore the basics of the Chinese herbal diagnostic system, you'll see that it goes beyond a simple one-to-one correlation.

Chinese herbal medicine uses a system that comes from a long history and tradition in China. The words, concepts, and system will seem different initially. Hang in there, and they will become familiar!

A HOLISTIC APPROACH

TCM and Chinese herbal medicine—like other traditional systems of medicine—look at the person as a whole, single unit. In modern Western medicine, you may have grown used to frequently seeing specialists, so you have a cardiologist for your heart, a therapist for your mental health, an orthopedist for your bones and joints, a dentist for your teeth, and an ophthalmologist for your eyes. You're essentially divided into sections.

In Chinese herbal medicine, the body and mind are one larger entity, and the systems in them work together, coordinate, and depend on the others for health, balance, and well-being. One system experiencing stress or imbalance can cause stress in others.

Another tenet of a holistic approach to healing involves identifying imbalances early in the disharmonizing process, before they worsen. It is so common for someone to come into a Chinese herbalist's office with symptoms they've tolerated for years, sometimes a decade or more. I had a patient who had suffered with constipation since the birth of her daughter 25 years earlier. We corrected the constipation and her skin issues in three to four months using Chinese herbal medicine. Holistic medicine works best when you are in tune with your body; for example, when you realize that for the past month there's been a tendency to constipation, it can be addressed while it's new and more easily resolved.

Take trouble falling asleep as another example. Chinese herbal medicine would not simply prescribe a sedating and calming herb. It looks at what imbalances are causing the sleep problems and addresses any underlying patterns. The treatment could include sedating and calming herbs while addressing the underlying causes, but after a period of time the herbs would not be needed anymore.

HARMONY

Chinese medicine, like Ayurveda and other traditional systems of medicine, uses nature as the ideal of harmony and cooperation. Like the steady shifts between seasons, the balance of predator and prey, and their reliance upon each other as members of an ecosystem, nature has a way of correcting disharmony and imbalance. Like humans who enter an ecosystem and disrupt it, your body, mind, and spirit are unhealthy when you are out of harmony and balance.

The words and descriptions used in Traditional Chinese Medicine are based on nature and this idea of harmony and cooperation. Concepts can be hard to describe without also explaining what intertwines and balances them. An excellent example of this is the concept of Yin and Yang.

YIN, YANG, AND BALANCE

We are made up of both Yin and Yang energetics, and in health they present in equal amounts. The energetic of Yin represents your ability to rest and be still, while Yang energy represents your ability to move and act. As you age, you can experience imbalances in Yin and Yang, with menopause and the hormonal shifts of late middle age representing two of the biggest shifts in amounts of and balance between the two energies. For many women, menopause is a time of lowered amounts of Yin, with menopausal symptoms relieved by correcting the imbalance and building Yin. The energy of Yin and Yang is stored in the kidneys, with Yin being housed in the left kidney and Yang in the right.

The white part of the circle represents Yang: energy, movement, sunlight, and force. It gives warmth and movement and circulation and lifts you up. Healthy Yang gives you energy during the day. Herbs that tonify or build Yang are hot to warm in temperature and are energizing. A prime example of a Yang tonic is Rou gui (cinnamon bark); it is heating and inspires movement and circulation.

The tiny dot of Yin (black) in the white background of Yang reminds you not to go too far and to keep your Yang energy grounded in Yin.

Yin represents moonlight, coolness, fluidity, and rest. It is the full, well-maintained radiator that keeps your body from overheating. Healthy Yin lets you rest well at night and sleep soundly without waking up and ensures that your skin, hair, and body in general are not dry. It represents your ability to embrace periods of rest or alone time. It balances the outward nature of Yang with inward, receptive qualities. The herbs that build Yin are warm to cool in temperature. They help you feel settled and at home in yourself and able to relax. While not immediately energizing like Yang tonics, they build your reserves for sustained activity and longevity. Two examples of Yin-building herbs are Tian men dong (asparagus root) and Mai men dong (ophiopogon).

The tiny dot of Yang in the Yin reminds you, again, not to go too far and to balance the internal qualities of Yin with the external.

Both Chinese and Western herbal medicine strive to do the same thing—to balance and improve health.

Both arose as traditional systems of medicine, with the roots of Western herbalism in ancient Greece.

Both systems have a framework-rooted in nature and elements, and both categorize herbs by temperature and taste (see The Qualities of Herbs on page 17).

Western herbalism often favors using "simples," or one single herb by itself. Chinese herbal medicine is based on the use of formulas, which are groups of herbs that work together like a musical composition. Each herb in the formula has a specific role for how it works and interacts with the other herbs. Some Chinese herbal formulas can have 12 to 18 ingredients, while Western herbal medicine formulas usually contain fewer herbs.

Today, the two systems are interacting with each other, with Western herbalists learning about Chinese diagnostic techniques and Chinese herbalists incorporating alcohol-based tinctures and local herbs.

An Approach to Illness and the Body

We will now dive deeper into the framework of Chinese herbal medicine to see how it describes health and identifies imbalances. Chinese herbal practitioners do not use Western medical terminology. Each system of the body, each energetic system, is assessed for health or imbalance. With a Chinese herbalist, an intake could take up to two hours and covers body temperature, emotions, bowel movements, diet, sleep, energy levels, and more.

THE BODY: ESSENCE, SPIRIT, QI, BLOOD, AND MOISTURE

In addition to Yin and Yang, you are made up of Essence, Spirit, Qi, Blood, and Moisture (Jin Ye). All of these substances, these smaller systems, work in harmony to keep you in balance. A weakness in one can affect the others.

Essence

Essence, or Jing, is your genetic inheritance. It is what you are born with and have to work with during your life. It is what makes you uniquely *you* and helps you express your gifts to the world. While you cannot change your Jing, you can work to protect and support it by keeping Yin and Yang balanced in the body and by observing healthy lifestyle habits overall. Any herb supports Jing if it addresses or maintains harmony in the body.

Spirit

Spirit, or Shen, resides in your Heart and travels through the body like blood circulating. An often-told story about Shen compares it to birds whose nest is in the Heart. For them to be present, centered, and rested, their nest must be a soft, comfortable, nourishing place. The Shen needs Blood, Yin, and Qi in sufficient quantities to rest well in the Heart.

Herbs that help with Shen fall into many categories. One example is He huan pi (albizzia peel), which calms Shen. Yuan zhi (polygala) and Long yan rou (longan) support the Shen by making sure there is sufficient Heart Blood to keep the nest for the Shen birds comfortable.

Qi

Qi (pronounced "chee") is the day-to-day energy you use to power your life, work, projects, and passions. The most common complaint I hear in practice is that of low energy and feeling tired. Modern societies often overspend and overdraw from their Qi bank accounts: That explains the popularity of coffee and energy drinks! Symptoms of low, depleted Qi include feeling tired and sleepy, with low motivation to do things like cook a nutritious meal for yourself instead of ordering takeout. Feeling weak or heavy, experiencing poor digestion, and (in severe cases) prolapsed organs can all be attributed to a lack of Qi to keep your systems energized.

The Spleen and Stomach, the energetic systems of the Earth element, make your Qi or energy that flows through your meridians. The Spleen and Stomach are like the power station that generates the energy you need for daily activities. I have yet to see a patient who didn't benefit from some amount of Spleen Qi supplementation. Sufficient Yang supports Qi, and when you deplete Qi for long enough, you can begin to deplete Yang.

Blood

In Chinese herbal medicine, Blood is different from the substance you are familiar with from Western medicine. Blood is an energetic concept like Qi or Shen. Healthy Yin nourishes and supports healthy Blood. If you deplete your Blood, eventually you will draw on Yin and begin depleting that as well. Just as Qi has common qualities with Yang, Blood has common qualities with Yin.

Moisture

Moisture, or Jin Ye, is the normal fluids in your body in proper balance. These fluids promote health through functions like lubricating joints, keeping our mucus membranes like lips and nose moist, and keeping synovial and cerebrospinal fluids in equilibrium.

THE FIVE ELEMENTS

ELEMENT	ASSOCIATED ORGANS
FIRE	Heart, Small Intestine, Triple Heater, Pericardium
EARTH	Stomach, Spleen
METAL	Lung, Large Intestine
WATER	Kidney, Bladder
WOOD	Liver, Gallbladder

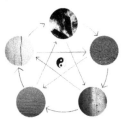

In Chinese herbal medicine, the macrocosm and microcosm—Mother Nature and your body—are made up of the Five Elements: Fire, Earth, Metal, Water, and Wood. They work together, balancing and building upon one another.

Each element corresponds to an energetic organ system. When Chinese herbal medicine refers to organs, it doesn't mean the physical organ. For example, in this book we'll talk about the Liver, but that doesn't mean your physical liver has an imbalance. Think of the Liver as an energetic system that includes the meridians or acupuncture channels that travel along your body as well as the physical and energetic properties of that organ system.

Fire

We lead off with Fire—the element of warmth, relationships and joy, and communication and connection to others. The Fire element corresponds to four organs instead of two: the Heart, Small Intestine, Pericardium, and Triple Heater. Three are physical organs as well, but the Triple Heater is a uniquely Chinese concept.

- The Heart is the Yin, the Emperor, who holds presence and acts as the center for all the other organ systems. Like the drummer in a band, it holds the rhythm and keeps everyone together and in harmony.

- The Small Intestine is the Yang pair to the Heart. It is the sorter, deciding what can be used and what should be filtered out.

- The Pericardium is also known as the Heart Protector and guards how close we let others in and who gets all the way into the Heart.

- The Triple Heater (known by many other names, including San Jiao) keeps you regulated in many ways, from physical temperature to emotional temperature. It can be described as homeostasis. Think about the Triple Heater when you've been at work talking to others all day, making presentations, and being engaged. Often, you need a break and some downtime. This is the balance of the Triple Heater—being extroverted, for some more than others, can take energy. These people need time alone to recharge. The physical aspects of the San Jiao or Triple Heater are also divided into areas of the body: upper, middle, and lower. The Upper Jiao is the chest. The Middle Jiao is the middle third of the body, including the torso and all the organs in the abdomen. The Lower Jiao is the lower abdomen.

Earth

Earth is the element of nourishment and sympathy, of caring for the self and others. In some ancient models, the Earth was at the center, with the other four elements circling around it. That is because some theorized that the Earth element was a foundation of the others, similar to how the Earth is home to the other four elements. The Earth element corresponds to the Stomach as the Yang organ and to the Yin Spleen energy systems. It is the center of the body, digestion, and processing. It is the powerhouse for the body, because the energy or Qi we use every day is produced by the Stomach and Spleen. Good digestion is the basis for good health. In my practice, the first formula every patient gets addresses digestive strength, to begin with the Earth element and to make the digestion of other herbs possible. When someone suffers from chronic low energy, the Earth element is top of the list for support.

Metal

Metal is the element of recognition, quality, inspiration, grief, and letting go. The Yin organ of Metal is the Lungs, and the Large Intestine is the Yang. A healthy Metal element can give and receive recognition and grieve and let go when it is appropriate. The Lungs breathe in physically but also help with metaphorical inspiration and are responsible for bringing in things and ideas of value and quality. The Large Intestine helps hold on to what is valuable, like nutrients, on a physical level, and lets go of what isn't serving or is no longer needed.

Water

The Water element is our foundation and sense of security and reserves. It is the source of our willpower, depth, fear, and wisdom. The Yin organ of Water is the Kidney, and the Yang is the Bladder. It is our sense of safety in the world and a healthy sense of fear. An imbalanced Water type could be a daredevil who has little or no fear and puts themselves in reckless, dangerous situations. On the other end of the spectrum, it could be a person who is always afraid and never takes chances. A healthy Water type would be balanced between the two, able to assess risk and manage fears. The Water element in balance has direction and a sense of purpose and is able to go with the flow.

Wood

The Wood element gives us direction and a vision of where we are headed and our place in the larger world. The Yin organ is the Liver, paired with the Yang Gallbladder. The Liver is the General. It knows the way forward and is ready to lead us there, getting the other organs to come along. While the Heart is royalty, the Liver is on the field, leading the way. The Yang Gallbladder helps us sort through choices and make decisions. The Gallbladder relies on the vision of the Liver to decide how to get us to our goal. Out of balance, we may lose hope, be unable to see a way forward, or be indecisive.

The Liver has been nicknamed the General, because it is responsible for schedules and leads the way. Energetically, a healthy Liver is working not just for the good of itself but for others. The gift of Wood is benevolence. Out of balance, the Wood element can be too controlling or caught up in details and can't see the bigger picture.

ILLNESS FACTORS

In addition to using Chinese herbal medicine to build up health by increasing Qi, Blood, Yin, and Yang, we can also use it to clear excessive conditions that promote imbalance. These excessive causes of illness include being too hot or too cold and building up the wrong type of fluids.

Heat and Cold

Heat and Cold are easy concepts, because we experience them daily. Too much Cold can damage Qi and Yang. For example, the Spleen (our Qi power source) doesn't like too much Cold, especially cold food. Heat can damage Blood and Yin in the way too much hot and spicy food can damage Stomach Yin and cause heartburn, indigestion, and other complaints. A warm herb like Xiao hui xiang (fennel) treats cold conditions, and a cold herb like Huang bai (skullcap) clears Heat.

I once had a client who lived in Hawaii for a few years. She loved soaking up the afternoon sun on the beach, but eventually she got too hot. She had depleted her Yin, causing dry skin and hair, extreme thirst, and, most problematic, insomnia with hot flashes and sweating at night. A formula that helped replenish her Yin and clear the Heat that had built up helped, along with buying a beach umbrella and going to the beach later in the evening when it was cooler and the sun wasn't as strong. Her sleep and Heat symptoms got increasingly better with the formula and lifestyle changes.

Dampness and Phlegm

Dampness and Phlegm are similar but have key differences and exist on a spectrum. Both are fluids that appear when we are out of balance, unlike Jin Ye, which indicates balance and proper functioning. Dampness and Phlegm are fluids showing up when and where they shouldn't. Phlegm is Dampness that stays around and doesn't get drained or moved out. Adding Heat or Cold can further congeal it into a thicker, stickier fluid that is then harder to drain or move. Dampness can be a runny nose after a meal or other clear fluid discharges. Phlegm is a benign cyst that forms under the skin or sinus congestion that begins to thicken and turn colors like yellow or green.

An herb like Fu ling (poria) drains Dampness. Phlegm is treated with slightly different herbs that are up to the task, including Xuan fu hua (inula flower).

Dampness and Phlegm are common because of how prevalent Spleen Qi weakness is in modern society. Many Spleen Qi building herbs will also help take care of Dampness, because the Spleen is responsible for getting fluids where they're supposed to be in health.

Wind

Wind is one of the more challenging concepts, because it is so different from any Western diagnosis. There are two kinds of Wind—Internal and External.

To start, imagine a windy day in autumn. Dry leaves are swirling and skidding along the sidewalk as the trees sway. Your hair flies around, and you feel the strong gusts. That night, you have a cough and a tickle in your throat—the beginnings of a cold, perhaps? This is the idea of External Wind, or catching a cold or cough. It enters through our most exterior energy meridians in the neck, throat, and head. Many people report feeling that tickle or sore throat at the beginning of a cold. In Chinese herbal medicine, the idea is to release that back to the exterior, or "kick it out," in a sense.

To explain Internal Wind, imagine a water hose that is clean, with no blockages and a full stream of water flowing through it. There isn't a lot of space in the hose, because the water is filling it up. Now imagine that there isn't enough liquid to fill the hose and it's only a third full. There is a lot of space for air in that hose. Air and wind can travel in that space. Inside your body, your vessels should be full of Yin and Blood, with no space for Wind to travel. With Blood and Yin deficiency, when there isn't enough to keep the vessels full, Wind can use those to move around. Most Internal Wind symptoms occur in the head and upper body, because wind likes to move upward. Common issues caused by

Internal Wind are migraine headaches and dizziness and vertigo. In Chinese herbal medicine, there are herbs like Gou teng (cat's claw) that anchor Internal Wind while Blood and Yin can be replenished.

Emotions

Chinese medicine views every emotion as appropriate in the correct situation. There are times in which anger, sadness, and grief are appropriate and should not be viewed as "bad" or "wrong."

Emotions can become a cause of illness when you get stuck in them and cannot move to other emotions when appropriate. Having sufficient time to process an emotion like grief is vital, but there should be a point at which the grief can move to allow room for other emotions.

There are no specific herbs to help with emotions. It depends on the emotion and the situation. However, when emotions are stuck, Qi is often stuck as well, and restoring flow helps balance it all out.

Chinese herbs are categorized by taste and temperature. They are further categorized by their energetic direction and the organs and channels they affect. (In chapter 3, you'll notice that this information is associated with each of the herbs listed.)

Temperature works along a spectrum: Hot > Warm > Neutral > Cool > Cold. Herbs that augment Yang are warm to hot. Herbs that clear Heat are cool to cold.

In Chinese herbal medicine, there are five tastes: sweet, sour, bitter, acrid, and salty. Herbs can have more than one flavor; most have two to three.

SWEET is a flavor we are all familiar with and the most palatable of the five. In Chinese herbal medicine, the sweet flavor tonifies, builds, and supplements. It is associated with the Earth element.

SOUR is rare, and its role is more of an astringent, toning and tightening to prevent the loss of fluids. It corresponds to the Wood element.

BITTER is a very common medicinal flavor and is found in the majority of Chinese herbs. Overall, the bitter flavor is draining and cooling. The modern American diet tends to shy away from the bitter flavor, but it holds an important place in maintaining health and balance. Bitter is associated with the Fire element.

ACRID is releasing, and many acrid-tasting herbs contain essential oils and aromatics. This flavor is found the most in the herbs that help release Exterior Wind (i.e., that cold we've caught at the office). Most plants that taste acrid contain aromatic essential oils that contribute to their strong, moving flavors. Examples are herbs like Du huo (angelica) and some mints and foods like green onions and cilantro leaves. Acrid corresponds to the Metal element.

SALTY is the least common flavor found in Chinese herbs. The salty flavor excels at breaking up nodules and dispersing accumulations. An example is Hai zao (sargassum), a seaweed. The salty flavor corresponds to the Water element.

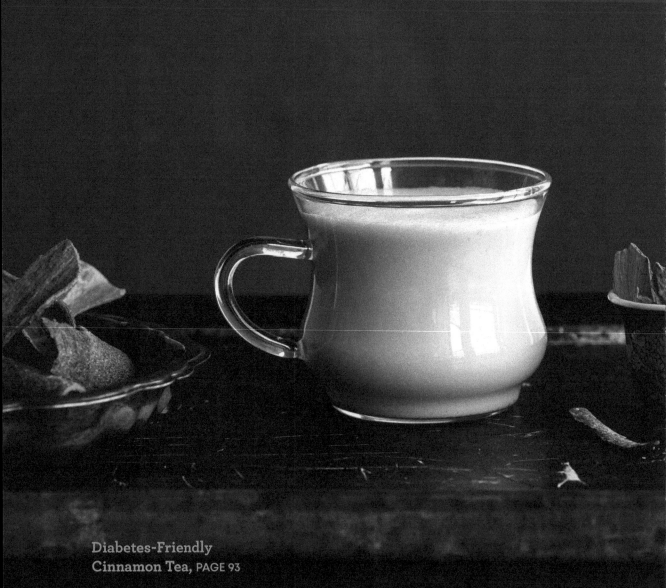

Diabetes-Friendly
Cinnamon Tea, PAGE 93

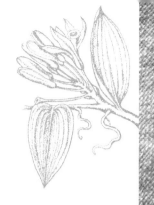

CHAPTER 2

Your Herbal Apothecary

In this chapter, you will learn the basics of making Chinese herbal medicine. We'll dive into the practical aspects of curating your herbal apothecary: what ingredients and equipment are most helpful, as well as the key methods for making Chinese herbal medicine. This chapter also includes growing and buying information, as well as tips for safety and best practices.

Diagnosis in Chinese Herbal Medicine

As we explore the herbs and formulas for your home apothecary, remember that there is no one answer for any ailment. A condition such as insomnia can have different causes depending on the person and their specific imbalance. In a Chinese herbal medicine practice, each formula is tailored to an individual and their individual needs. This means that the remedies and formulas provided in part III are guides that can be modified using what you know about Chinese herbal medicine to be your personal remedy for your unique needs.

Getting Started with Your Home Apothecary

One way to start a home apothecary is to decide which herbs and formulas are best for you and begin to gather those ingredients. It is also helpful to look at the upcoming season and what you might need in the near future: In other words, have your spring allergy formula or winter cold remedy ready before you need it.

Throughout the centuries of Chinese herbal medicine, formulas have been based on decoctions of dried herbs. This is great news for the beginner, because making a decoction is an easy but effective way to get started. It does not require a large investment or a complicated setup (see Herbal Decoctions on page 24).

WHERE TO BUY

Online shopping gives you so many choices, but with those options comes the responsibility to gather information and make an informed purchase.

The best practice is to buy your dried herbs from a company that is transparent about how the herb is grown (organic or without pesticides) and how it is harvested. Quality companies will provide all of this information for customers (for a list of reputable companies, see Resources, page 187). Sustainable growing and harvesting are vital to ensure a healthy supply of that herb in the future. If you find a local apothecary or herb shop, ask questions and support them if the quality is good. Can they tell you where the herbs they carry were sourced? Is the botanical name available? I once went into a local herb shop that listed two different plants as the same when they had different botanical names and slightly different usage. That worried me, and I ended up not purchasing from them. For safety and quality purposes, you need to know exactly what you are buying.

An example is American ginseng (Xi yang shen). This native American herb has been wild harvested to dangerously low levels. Poaching is a problem in many areas, and the herb's survival is threatened by irresponsible overharvesting. It is now cultivated on farms, but it is a challenging crop that can take up to a decade to be ready for harvest. In response to the dwindling supply, the price has gone up, and it is neither an affordable nor a sustainable herb to buy responsibly.

Always know what form of herbs you are purchasing. When buying bulk dried herbs, you might be given an option for powdered or cut and sifted pieces that look chopped. What you purchase will depend on how long you want to store it and what you're doing with it—for example, whether you're making capsules or decocting the herb with water.

Premade Herbal Formulas

Regulations for quality control of premade, packaged Chinese herbal formulas vary by country, and the safest products are those you can verify have been produced using GMP. GMP stands for Good Manufacturing Processes and ensures a level of safety and consistency in manufacturing. Products will also be clearly labeled if they have been grown organically or tested for pesticides and heavy metals. If you are buying a product produced by an American, Australian, European, or Canadian company, it will have a GMP label on the bottle. Some herbal apothecaries prefer to sell to practitioners and may ask for a license before purchase. (More information on formulas can be found in chapter 4.)

Many herbal suppliers also carry containers in a variety of sizes and materials for storing your herbal medicines.

WHAT TO GROW

Growing Chinese medicinal herbs outside of China and in the United States is gaining popularity. What you can grow depends on where you live and your available space. Both China and the United States are large countries that contain a range of growing zones. As Chinese medicinal herbs are less common than Western herbs, it is easier to procure seeds than live plants for starting a Chinese herbal medicine garden.

My favorite company that truly understands growing medicinal herbs is Strictly Medicinal, based in Oregon. They sell seeds from all traditions of herbal medicine, including Western, Ayurvedic, and Chinese. The seeds and plants they sell are listed with Pinyin, botanical, and common names. Richo Cech, whose family founded Strictly Medicinal, includes valuable insight on the plants and experience on growing from seed. Some live plants are also available.

For a six-ingredient Starter's Garden that includes some of the easier herbs to grow, you could try:

- Xiao hui xiang (fennel)
- Hu lu ba (fenugreek)
- Yi mu cao (motherwort)
- Ai ye (mugwort)
- Gou qi zi (goji berry)
- Huang qi (astragalus)

Strictly Medicinal has a Chinese Medicinal Herb Seed Collection, but they have more Chinese herbs than just that collection. Some of the herbs or seeds they have for purchase are:

- Dan shen (salvia)
- Dang shen (codonopsis)
- Huang qin (skullcap)
- Xu duan (dipsacus)
- Yi mu cao (motherwort)
- Ku shen (sophora root)
- Wu wei zi (schisandra)
- Mai men dong (ophiopogon)
- Chuan xin lian (andrographis)
- Bai shao (white peony)
- Chi shao (red peony)
- Huo xiang (agastache)

In addition, there are some Western varieties that are similar enough to their Chinese counterparts that you can interchange them. One example is Sheng ma (black cohosh). Western and Chinese herbalists use types of black cohosh that are different cultivars but function very similarly to each other. A Chinese herbalist could use the Western black cohosh and get similar results as with the imported Chinese Sheng ma.

HERBAL MEDICINE AND ACUPUNCTURE

When you read this book and discover you have a few of the patterns and could use some herbs to help with balance, you will find that if you go to an acupuncturist, you will be treated for those same imbalances. Finding the patterns of disharmony is a foundation for all of the treatment modalities in Chinese medicine. In addition to acupuncture, practitioners can determine whether moxibustion, tui na, and cupping will also support the work that Chinese herbal medicine offers. The effects are cumulative, and all the techniques of TCM work together to help restore balance.

KEY INGREDIENTS AND HELPFUL EQUIPMENT

While the most common way to extract or prepare Chinese herbs is with water, some remedies will use other ingredients such as alcohol or oil to extract or molasses to preserve the herbs.

- High-quality oil like almond, coconut, olive, or sesame
- Beeswax
- Cloth for compresses
- Alcohol
- Molasses

Much of the equipment required for Chinese herbal medicine is already part of a well-appointed kitchen. Here's my list of essentials:

- Bowls of multiple sizes (small to medium, glass or stainless steel preferred)
- Blender or coffee grinder
- Coffee press or teapot (for infusions)
- Stockpot that can hold more than 9 cups of water and is *not* aluminum—stainless steel, ceramic, and glass are excellent options
- Food scale
- Glass containers
- Measuring cups
- Mortar and pestle (I prefer marble)
- Plastic dish basin for soaks
- Pyrex measuring cups in 2-cup and 8-cup sizes
- Slow cooker
- Strainers, small and large
- Tea bags (empty, plastic-free if possible)
- Teakettle

ADAPT WHAT YOU HAVE

The equipment listed is useful, but this isn't meant to be an exercise in shopping for a lot of kitchen gadgets. For home use, the purpose of the blender/coffee grinder and mortar and pestle is to break down big pieces into smaller pieces. This could also be done with a towel and a rolling pin! If you have large pieces of dried herbs and you need them to be smaller pieces, try running them through your blender, chopping them with a knife, or even breaking them by hand.

You can also adapt whatever you have on hand for storage. While I love my 8-cup Pyrex measuring cup with lid, I already had it when I realized it was perfect for storing herbal decoctions. You may have a piece in your kitchen that wasn't designed for Chinese herbal medicine but can do the job quite nicely.

Methods and Brewing

Medicine-making in Chinese herbal medicine and medicine-making in Western herbal medicine have many similarities and some key differences. Western herbal medicine uses tinctures extensively. Tinctures use alcohol to extract the herbs for internal use. Many Western herbalists feel the strongest medicine is made by creating a tincture with fresh herbs at the time of harvest.

The most common Chinese herbal medicines are made using dried herbs that are extracted in water to make a decoction. Chinese herbal medicine has some use of alcohol in its history, but decoctions are valued as potent and effective.

HERBAL DECOCTIONS

Herbal decoctions are the most-used method for preparing Chinese herbal medicine formulas. A decoction uses water to extract medicinal constituents from the herbs. I consider them the strongest, most potent way to take herbs internally and have had patients who were not getting results with other forms of herbal medicine who had improvements as soon as they switched to decoctions.

To make a decoction, you will need:

- Herbs
- Large bowl
- Blender or grinder
- Strainer
- Large (non-aluminum) stockpot or slow cooker
- 8-cup glass measuring cup or similar size storage jar

A good way to make your decoction is by the week so that you can cook it on a day when you have more time and then keep seven days' worth in the refrigerator.

Place your herbs in a large bowl. If there are pieces larger than a quarter, chop them in a blender or grinder if possible.

<u>Method One:</u> Place your herbs in the stockpot and add enough water to cover the herbs by at least an inch. Bring it to a boil, then reduce the heat and simmer gently for 20 or 30 minutes. Check after 15 minutes to see whether the water is getting low and not completely covering the herbs. If needed, add more to cover the herbs. Remove the stockpot from the heat and cool.

<u>Method Two:</u> Place your herbs in the slow cooker and cover with at least an inch of water. Allow the herbs to decoct on the lowest setting for about eight hours or overnight. Check after 30 to 60 minutes to see whether more water is needed to cover the herbs completely. When cooking is complete, turn off the slow cooker and cool.

Place the strainer on your 8-cup Pyrex measuring cup or similar container, and pour the liquid into the bowl, leaving the herbs in the strainer. This is the herbal decoction you will drink. Refrigerate the liquid and discard the cooked herbs. (They are great in compost!) For a week of herbs, you want to end up with about seven cups of decocted herbal tea for a dose of half a cup twice a day, equaling one cup per day. If you end up with eight cups, divide what you have by seven and drink it over the week. If you end up with less than that, simply add water to bring the total up to seven cups. This is an inexact science, because different dried herbs absorb different amounts of water as they cook. After seven days, discard any remaining decoction and prepare your herbal formula for the following week.

Remember: Taste is part of the therapeutic value of Chinese herbal medicine. Many people grow used to the taste of their herbs. Some like to hold their nose and drink their dose fast to be done with it, while others prefer to water their dose down with a few more cups of hot water and drink it slowly throughout the day from a thermos or insulated mug.

INFUSIONS

Not used much in Chinese herbal medicine, an infusion is soaking rather than cooking herbs in water. If you are preparing one or two herbs alone and they are leaves or flowers, you can infuse them. If a formula contains more dense, heavy materials such as roots and twigs, they need to be decocted. Infusions are for lighter, more delicate herbal matter.

You will need:

- Herbs
- Coffee press
- Boiling water

Place your herbs in a coffee press and add boiling water. Allow the herbs to infuse for at least an hour. For a stronger infusion, leave the herbs to soak longer. One method is to allow them to infuse overnight to drink the next morning. Alternately, you can use a teapot instead of a coffee press and filter the herbs through a small strainer into a mug or a 2-cup glass measuring cup.

Infusions work well with daily doses of herbs as well as weekly formulas. If you infuse a weekly amount, strain it into a storage container and refrigerate.

SOAKS AND COMPRESSES

A soak or compress uses decocted herbs, so prepare the formula using the instructions for Herbal Decoctions (page 24).

After preparing the decoction, you will place the soak or compress on the area that needs it. Your skin is an organ that can absorb and "digest" herbs. Remember that these herbs have strong qualities, including color. Some, like Jiang huang (turmeric), temporarily leave an orange hue on the skin but can permanently stain clothing.

You will need:

- Cloth (a washcloth or absorbent cotton cloth)
- Herbal decoction (see page 24)
- Plastic dish basin or large plastic bowl
- Storage container

Soak the cloth in the warm herbal decoction and apply to the affected area. Wrapping in another cloth can help preserve the warmth.

If the pain is in the hand, wrist, foot, or ankle, you can soak the area directly in the herbal decoction. Plastic dish basins or a plastic bowl large enough for one or both of your feet are good options for soaks. Add enough warm water to the herbal decoction to cover the area to be soaked; also soak the compress cloth, wash the area to be soaked, and then soak for 15 to 30 minutes. Keep this decoction and use it again for up to five days. Mark the storage container clearly with "Herbal Soak" and that it is *not* for internal consumption. For use on subsequent days, warm the decoction before using.

With compresses, I often soak in the herbal decoction at the same time. For example, with knee pain, have the foot and ankle soaking in the herbal decoction while the compress is on the knee. I have also used herbal foot soaks with patients who were on multiple pharmaceuticals, making it prudent to avoid taking herbs orally. Compresses and herbal soaks can be very therapeutic.

Herbal soaks become herbal baths by simply soaking the entire body in the herbal decoction.

Eye Compresses

In Chinese herbal medicine, there are herbs that excel at treating eye conditions. You will learn about them in chapter 3.

You will need:

- 2 empty tea bags (preferably plastic-free)
- Herbs
- Large mug
- Bowl

Fill the empty tea bags with the herbs. Put the filled tea bags in the mug, pour boiling water over, and infuse for 20 minutes.

Transfer the tea bags to a bowl and drink the infusion. Once the teabags have cooled, sit back and relax with one herbal tea bag on each closed eye.

CAPSULES

Capsules and capsule-making machines for home use are inexpensive and easy to find. They vary somewhat in the parts they contain and specific instructions, but a capsule machine gives you a way to hold a large number of capsules open, fill them all with herbal material, and close them.

For capsules you need powdered herbs. Herbs can be purchased powdered, or you can powder dried herbs in a coffee grinder. It takes time and a powerful blender to get particles small enough for capsules.

You will need:

- Capsule machine
- Empty capsules in the correct size
- Powdered herbs
- Large bowl
- Baking sheet or aluminum foil
- Small bowl
- Spoon
- Dry, clean cloth
- Jar for storing finished, filled capsules

Read the instructions for your specific machine and make sure you have the correct size capsules to fill it. I use a Cap M Quik machine, but there are other quality brands like The Capsule Machine.

In a large bowl, mix the powdered herbs thoroughly to get even distribution. Put the bowl aside and place the baking sheet or aluminum foil under your capsule machine.

Separate the empty capsules, placing the bottom halves into the capsule machine and the tops into the small bowl. Once you've filled the capsule machine with the bottoms, place the small bowl of tops aside.

Keep in mind that machines vary, so add or remove steps specific to your capsule machine. With a spoon, fill the capsules with the herbs from the large bowl. Using the tamper that comes with your machine, tamp down the herbs inside the capsules, then add more. Repeat, filling and tamping until you have filled them as much as possible. Push the tops onto the bottoms.

Holding the dry cloth in one hand, remove the capsules from the machine and gently wipe any extra powdered herbs from the outside of the capsules. Then place them in the storage jar.

Return any powdered herbs that have fallen onto the baking sheet to the large bowl and start the process again, repeating until you've encapsulated your herbal formula. Clearly label your jar with the date and the name of your formula, including a list of all the herbs in it.

The benefits of capsules are that you can travel with them and the taste is neutralized. Herbal formulas are designed for their health benefit and almost always contain herbs that are not sweet but bitter or acrid. However, digestion starts in the tongue, and many herbalists believe that the taste of the herbs is part of the medicine. The downsides with capsules are that you can't taste them, and making them is time-consuming, detail-oriented work.

Remember your capsule size (e.g., 0, 00) because this determines your dosage.

GRANULES OR GRANULAR HERBS

Granules are incredibly popular with Chinese herbalists. Different from powdered herbs, these are herbs that have been cooked into a concentrated herbal decoction, then dried into tiny granules about the size of coarse polenta. This is where herbal decoctions meet modern technology. Granules are single herbs or formulas concentrated to a strength ranging from 5 times to 12 times stronger than a simple at-home decoction. This potency will be listed on the bottle and in the company's information and will be listed with the granule strength first. An example is 5:1, meaning the granules are five times the strength of a decoction. Granules are most often sold only to practitioners with a license. I'm including them here to differentiate them from dried herbs that are powdered, as mentioned in the Capsules section (page 27).

Granules dissolve in very hot water, allowing them to be prepared quickly. Since they are dry until water is added, they are as easy to travel with as capsules while retaining the flavor of the herbal formula. Granules are a great option for those who simply cannot commit to cooking an herbal formula or need a more transportable form.

LINIMENTS

A liniment uses alcohol to extract the medicinal qualities of herbs. They are topical remedies for aches and pains. Chinese herbal liniments go beyond simple analgesics used for relieving pain; the herbs in liniment formulas treat the underlying patterns of disharmony to help heal and repair the injury or the cause of pain. Often, pain is a result of stagnation of Qi or Blood or both. An injury that doesn't properly heal can cause further pain in the future, making liniments an important remedy to have in your home apothecary.

You will need:

- Herbs
- Glass container or jar with lid
- Vodka or similar-strength alcohol
- Small strainer

Place the herbs in the glass jar, leaving at least two inches between the top of the herbs and the lid of the jar. Fill the jar to the top with alcohol, making sure it completely covers the herbs, then secure the lid. Allow the herbs to soak in the alcohol for at least six weeks, storing in a cool spot out of direct sunlight, and shaking it daily (or as often as you remember) to mix all the ingredients. After six weeks have passed, strain the herbs from the alcohol and store the liniment in a glass container out of the sun.

Liniments are excellent topical treatment for pain, injuries, and bruising. They are not meant to be taken internally. While alcohol excels at extracting and preserving the medicinal qualities of herbs, liniments must be applied frequently for best results.

OILS

Infused oils use an oil to extract the medicinal qualities of herbs. There are many different oils to choose from, and they all have different smells and textures on the skin. Just as herbs have specific properties, so do oils—for example, coconut oil is more cooling, and sesame oil is more warming—but in the end, you should choose the oil you like and will be happy to use on your skin. Some herbal suppliers will also carry these oils.

You will need:

- Glass container with lid

- Herbs

- Oil of your choice: almond, coconut, sesame, olive

- Small strainer

- Glass container for storing finished infused oil

Fill the glass container with the herbs, leaving space between the top of the herbs and the top of the jar. Cover completely with the oil and secure the lid. It is important that no herbs are above the oil and remain uncovered, as this can ruin the oil. Place your jar of herbs and oil in a cool, dark location and keep it there for six weeks, then strain and store in a glass container. Refrigeration after infusion is recommended, and oils should always be kept away from heat to protect them from going rancid.

OINTMENTS

Ointments are infused herbal oils thickened with beeswax.

You will need:

- 1 ounce (or 2 tablespoons) beeswax pellets or pastilles

- 8 ounces (or 1 cup) infused herbal oil (see page 29)

- Double boiler setup (a bowl over water in a slow cooker or a bowl over water in a pot on the stovetop)

- Spoon

- Spatula

- Storage container of choice (tin or glass are common choices); for example, five 2-ounce tin containers or three 4-ounce tin or glass containers

Place the beeswax and infused herbal oil in a bowl and place over the bowl of water on your heat source—either a slow cooker or the stovetop. Melt over low heat, and use a spoon to mix the two together. You want to heat them just enough to blend well. Remove from the heat source and use a spatula to transfer into your container.

Ointments keep for up to a year when kept cool and in a dark storage area.

SALVES

A salve is also made from infused herbal oil, but it has more beeswax than an ointment, giving it a more solid consistency.

You will need:

- Double boiler setup (a bowl over water in a slow cooker or a bowl over water in a pot on the stovetop) or crockpot

- 1 ounce (or 2 tablespoons) beeswax pellets or pastilles

- 4 ounces (or ½ cup) infused herbal oil (see page 29)

- Storage container of choice (tin or glass are common choices); for example, five 2-ounce tin containers or three 4-ounce tin or glass containers

Using a double boiler on the low setting on your stove or using a crockpot to ensure low temperatures, melt the beeswax by heating it with the infused herbal oil at a low temperature, mixing well. Immediately pour your warm mixture into the storage container.

Storage and Shelf Life

All herbal medicine, no matter the form, should be stored somewhere cool and dark. Oils go rancid, so products that are oil-based need refrigeration. Herbal bottles are tinted brown and blue, because sunlight degrades quality and shortens shelf life. With every herb you purchase and prepare, make sure to clearly mark it with its complete name and the date it was purchased or made. Keeping your herbs clearly marked is a must for safety and quality. When I imagine an apothecary, it involves shelves full of jars of herbs. While that is a wonderful way to store herbs (as long as the room doesn't get strong sun), it takes up a lot of space. When I don't have space for jars for each herb, I keep them in airtight, sealed bags marked with their names and purchase dates in a large storage tub. This ensures they do not attract pests and bugs.

Larger pieces retain their potency longer than smaller pieces or powders. When buying herbs and spices, the best practice is to buy larger pieces to grind, chop, or grate as needed. This is especially important for spices and aromatic herbs like mint that can quickly lose their potency. Roots can be stored longer than aerial parts. My policy is to keep roots that aren't powdered for up to two years and leafy aerial parts for a year. Using everything sooner rather than later is the best policy.

BEST PRACTICES

One of my previous positions was as supervisor of the Herb Clinic at the Academy for Five Element Acupuncture. At the beginning of every Herb Clinic residency, interns are trained in the school dispensary to ensure safety and accuracy when filling patient formulas. Here are some guidelines to bring these safety practices to your home apothecary:

- Keep your workspace clean. When working with herbs that you will ingest internally, use a food-grade cleaner on your counters.

- It bears repeating: Always mark everything clearly with a name and date and other pertinent information. I suspect every herbalist, at some point, has had a bottle or container of some herbal something that remained a mystery.

- Choosing how to store your herbs, oils, salves, liniments, and other creations is largely up to personal preference. I advise staying away from plastic as much as possible. Take time to look through what companies offer (e.g., sizes of tins for salves and ointments) to decide what you like and need.

Health care is a team effort, and while Chinese herbal medicine is a valuable team member, remember to go to your doctor and other health care team members for regular checkups. More doctors are becoming aware of the benefits of Chinese medicine, and they should know all the ways you are taking care of your health. If you are nervous about telling your doctor that you are using Chinese herbal medicine, my strategy is to go in with information to show why you chose to do so. Bring this book, have the full names of the herbs you are using, show any research you have, and tell them how you feel it is helping you. Similarly, you can always call a Chinese herbal practitioner with questions or concerns or for help deciding what herbs would be best for your particular situation.

Safety

Here are some safety precautions to keep in mind before you get started. Always know exactly what herb you are buying, and confirm botanical names and Chinese Pinyin names. A common name is not enough to identify an herb with absolute certainty.

Take your herbs at a different time from any medication you take, and make sure you've read the precautions for each herb and formula. If you are on a blood thinner like Coumadin, the therapeutic window is so small that I do not advise taking herbs internally while on this prescription.

In a perfect world, you would take your herbs on an empty stomach for maximum absorption. However, life can get busy. If the only way you can remember your herbs is to take them with a meal, go ahead and do so. It does make them slightly less effective, but it won't entirely negate their effect. Taking herbs with food is better than not taking them at all because your timing was off.

The most common interaction that I have seen between herbs and pharmaceuticals is mutual enhancement, meaning that they help each other. A patient taking a prescription for high blood pressure who starts taking herbs to help ease tension and calm the Shen may find their blood pressure decreases further. As you start Chinese herbal medicine, monitor yourself diligently and share that information with the rest of your health care team.

Let's Get Started!

Now it's time to dig in! If this feels overwhelming, take a deep breath. Find a few herbs you think can help you, and try preparing them. Herbal decoctions are a great place to start, because they are effective but also simple and a lot like other basic cooking. In the next chapter, you will learn more about 35 single herbs, and in chapter 4, you will discover how to combine these herbs into formulas and remedies.

Decoction for a Cold
with a Dry Cough, PAGE 104

Part Two

HERBS

This part is a simplified, shortened version of a Chinese herbal *Materia Medica* textbook. In this section, you'll learn about 35 different herbs. Here, you'll learn the common, Pinyin, and Latin names of the herbs as well as where they fit into the scope of Chinese herbal medicine diagnostics. You'll also find information on growing the herbs, if possible, and what to take into consideration when purchasing them.

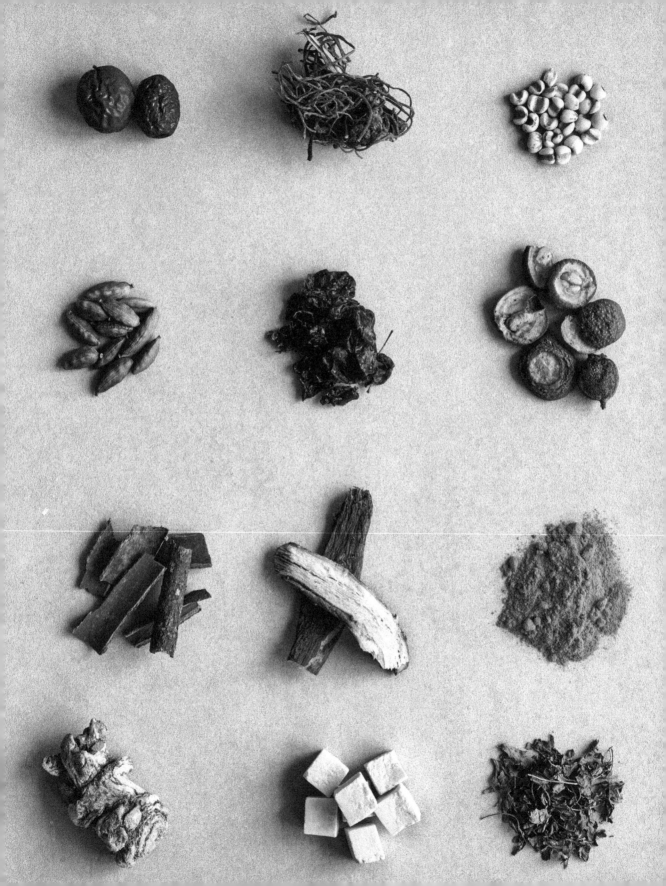

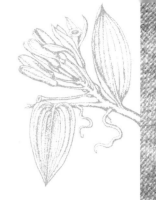

CHAPTER 3

Herb Profiles

This chapter contains profiles of 35 essential herbs and how they work according to Chinese medicinal principles. Each herb profile describes its temperature, treatment category, personality, and historical use, along with modern research where applicable. There are so many amazing herbs that it is a challenge to narrow it down to 35. The herbs listed here represent the diverse categories of Chinese herbal medicine, with a focus on herbs that are easier to source, inexpensive, and safer. I've included a few that you can even grow yourself. There is a saying among herbalists: You can know 50 herbs one way or one herb 50 ways. Knowing the herbs in this chapter will give you a solid foundation to cover many patterns of disharmony.

The layout of this chapter is different from a traditional, exhaustive *Materia Medica*. A Chinese *Materia Medica* can be overwhelming, with more than 1,000 pages and hundreds of herbs. They are also organized by treatment category, not alphabetically, and beginners struggle to navigate this format. This chapter is alphabetical by common name to be more approachable for the beginner but also includes the herb's Pinyin name and Latin name.

> **A Note about Pinyin**
> *Pinyin takes Chinese characters and spells them out phonetically with English letters. There are sites and apps that can help with pronunciation, and the Pinyin name is important for clarity in identifying the herb.*

Read through this chapter and get to know the herbs. Later, when you have a specific question about an herb or are trying a formula using a combination of herbs, you can use it as a reference to return to and review the information.

Herbs by Category

For ease of use, here's a list of herbs by category:

- **Tonify Qi:** Huang qi (astragalus), Bai zhu (atractylodes), Da zao (dates)

- **Tonify Blood:** Gou qi zi (goji), Sang shen (mulberry), Bai shao (peony)

- **Tonify Yin:** Tian men dong (asparagus root), Mai men dong (ophiopogon)

- **Tonify Yang:** Rou gui (cinnamon bark), Hu lu ba (fenugreek), Xu duan (teasel)

- **Regulate Qi:** Xiang fu (cyperus), Chen pi (tangerine peel), Mei gui hua (rosebud)

- **Regulate Blood:** Chuang xiong (ligusticum), Jiang huang (turmeric), Dan shen (salvia)

- **Calm the Shen:** He huan pi and He huan hua (albizzia), Long yan rou (longan), Ling zhi (reishi)

- **Clear Heat:** Mu dan pi (tree peony)

- **Warm the Interior:** Yi zhi ren (cardamom), Xiao hui xiang (fennel)

- **Cool, Acrid, Release External Wind:** Ju hua (chrysanthemum), Bo he (mint), Ge gen (kudzu)

- **Warm, Acrid, Release External Wind:** Gui zhi (cinnamon twig)

- **Anchor Interior Wind:** Gou teng (cat's claw)

- **Food Stagnation:** Shan zha (hawthorn)

- **Stabilize and Bind:**
  Shan zhu yu (cornus)

- **Transform Phlegm, Stop Coughing:** Zi wan (aster), Gua lou (tricosanthes fruit)

- **Expel Wind Dampness:**
  Du huo (angelica)

- **Drain Dampness:**
  Fu ling (poria), Yi yi ren (Job's tears)

ON TONICS

On the following pages, you'll discover herbs from 17 different categories. Many of them can be used as tonics. Because of their simplicity, beginners are often drawn first to tonics, the herbs that build you up. The Tonics category is divided into the following four parts:

- **Tonify Qi:** a Qi Tonic warms and builds Qi

- **Tonify Blood:** a Blood Tonic nourishes and builds Blood

- **Tonify Yin:** a Yin Tonic cools and nourishes Yin

- **Tonify Yang:** a Yang Tonic warms and builds Yang

Qi and Yang Tonics are warming, while Blood and Yin Tonics are overall cooling.

Determining exactly which of these qualities is lacking helps identify the appropriate type of herb to use as a tonic. Tonics also have some sweetness and therefore taste better and more familiar. Note that while tonic herbs are a gift from the plant world and we are lucky to have them, they sometimes work best with herbs that perform other functions.

A deficiency often occurs along with an excess, so a formula would be composed to build what is deficient and clear what is excess. For example, as you deplete your cooling Yin, Heat can begin to build. Classic Yin-tonifying formulas address both at the same time by combining Yin Tonics with herbs that clear Heat. Another example is Qi Tonics. As people suffer from insufficient Qi, they have trouble circulating Qi. As in a pipe that gets clogged when water flow is weak and material builds up, if there's not enough Qi flowing, things start to get stuck. Classic Qi Tonic formulas combine tonic herbs with herbs that move Qi and fluids. You will learn more about the elegance and balance of Chinese herbal formulas in chapter 4.

Joint pain that is caused by Wind Dampness has a special term: *Bi* (pronounced "bee"). This is pain that can come and go, change from day to day, and feel different depending on the weather. It may feel like stiffness more than sharp pain. Any cause of pain, such as an injury or trauma, that isn't cleared or brought back into balance can become worse and have other patterns compounding it, including Bi syndrome. For example, an injury like a bad sprain that isn't properly treated can leave weakness or imbalance in a joint, resulting in later pain from Bi Wind Dampness.

Albizzia • He huan pi (peel) and He huan hua (flower)

Albizziae julibrissinis cortex and *Albizziae julibrissinis flos*

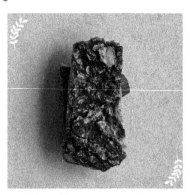

Parts used: peel and flower

As students, we called He huan pi (albizzia) happy bark, because *huan* translates as happy. Going to the Liver and Heart, both He huan pi (*pi* means peel) and He huan hua (*hua* means flower) calm the Shen, gently moving stagnant Qi to smooth out emotions and physical discomfort. Their temperature is neutral—not too warm and not too cool—and the flavor is sweet. The bark is stronger than the flower, but the flower is lovely and better tasting to some.

Albizzia grows easily in the United States, so much so that it is considered a weed and even an invasive species in some states. Weeds can be great medicines: They are easier to grow and have fewer challenges to supply than a more delicate or harder-to-cultivate medicinal like ginseng.

He huan pi is decocted, but the flower, He huan hua, is much lighter material and can be infused.

Note: If you choose to wild harvest, make sure you know the soil and growing conditions of the tree.

Angelica • Du huo
Angelicae pubescentis radix

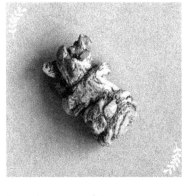

Part used: root

Warm, acrid, and bitter, Du huo (angelica) goes to the Kidney and Bladder and dispels Wind Dampness from the lower body. It can also be used for the body aches that come with a cold or flu.

Dampness is a cause of pain. Du huo treats Wind Cold Dampness Bi syndrome anywhere in the body but especially in the lower half, including the lower back, legs, knees, and feet.

Du huo can also be used as a topical mouth rinse for a toothache to help with pain relief.

Similar herbs: Yi yi ren (Job's tears), Ge gen (kudzu)

PRECAUTIONS: Du huo can worsen dryness and Yin deficiency. It's not to be confused with Dang gui (*Angelica sinensis*).

Asparagus Root • Tian men dong
Asparagi cochinensis tuber

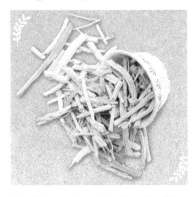

Part used: root

Tian men dong (asparagus root) is a Kidney and Lung Yin tonic and is very cold, sweet, and bitter. A Yin tonic for the whole body, it helps with symptoms of Kidney Yin deficiency like slight dizziness, tinnitus (the kind that stays around all the time), urine that is a darker yellow, dry mouth and thirst (especially at night), and a sore back. Its moisture and support for fluids mean it can help with dry constipation, a dry cough, and vaginal dryness. As it builds Yin in the Heart, it cools, clearing Heat and irritability.

Tian men dong is very similar to shatavari, one of the most used and respected herbs in Ayurvedic herbal medicine.

Similar herbs: Mai men dong (ophiopogon)

PRECAUTIONS: As a Yin tonic, this contains very sweet and dense materials, making it hard to digest; use with herbs for digestion like Chen pi (tangerine peel) or Xiao hui xiang (fennel) if needed.

Aster • Zi wan
Asteris tatarici radix

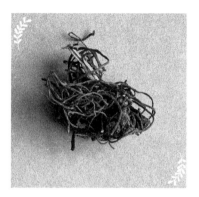

Part used: root

Zi wan (aster) can transform Phlegm and stop coughing.

One of the worst parts of having a cold or flu is the cough that lingers long after the rest of the symptoms have cleared. Zi wan is incredibly useful for clearing mucus and alleviating coughs. Neither too hot nor too cold, it is excellent for both chronic coughs and coughs that accompany a cold or flu.

Scientists have researched the traditional uses of Zi wan and agree that it is effective as an expectorant and antitussive as well as being anti-inflammatory.

Similar herbs: Gua lou (tricosanthes)

Growing: Both seeds and plants are available in the United States. It is a beautiful purple flower you can grow easily in your yard or garden.

Astragalus • Huang qi
Astragali membranacei radix

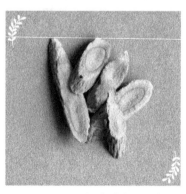

Part used: root

Huang qi (astragalus) is one of three Spleen and Lung Qi tonic herbs included in this truncated *Materia Medica*, but it is unique in its lifting, upward qualities that earn it the nickname of the "antigravity" herb. It goes beyond Bai zhu (atractylodes) in that it supports the Spleen Qi but also lifts and supports deficient Spleen Yang, which presents as a low, sinking, exhausted feeling and frequently needing to sit down.

Slightly warming, Huang qi can stop sweating and generate new flesh (like with wounds that are slow to heal and the production of new skin and tissue) and has become known for its help with immunity. Research in pharmacology shows that Huang qi is an antioxidant that cools inflammation, regulates the immune system, lowers cholesterol and blood sugar, protects the liver, and can be a useful, supportive herb in preventing cancer and assisting during cancer treatment.

Spleen Qi tonics and herbs in general often help with blood-sugar management. Akin to very healthy foods, herbs are beneficial to your body in the same way as eating vegetables and whole foods. But they feature extra qualities that help even more. In ancient China, people were unaware of the pancreas and attributed all of its functions to the Spleen. You will even see some texts that refer to it as the Spleen/Pancreas for this reason. Spleen Qi tonics support digestion and blood sugar and can have a positive influence on conditions like prediabetes.

Sweet like most tonic herbs, its flavor is not overwhelming, and it can be used in daily cooking for its many health benefits.

<u>Similar herbs:</u> Bai zhu (atractylodes), Da zao (dates)

PRECAUTIONS: As a Qi tonic it is warming and drying, so be cautious with Heat or insufficient Yin. It can lower blood sugar; monitor your levels with your doctor if you are diabetic.

Atractylodes • Bai zhu
Atractylodis macrocephalae rhizoma

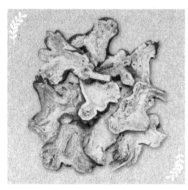

<u>Part used:</u> root

Bai zhu (atractylodes) is the steadfast, dependable workhorse of Chinese herbal medicine. Ginseng and mushrooms get the attention and fame, but Bai zhu deserves recognition as well. Inexpensive and one of the most frequently used herbs for tonifying Spleen and Lung Qi, it is found in dozens of formulas.

The Spleen is responsible for making the daily Qi, for taking the food and herbs we ingest and converting them into energy. It manages and transports fluids. When the Spleen Qi is weak, fluids will become imbalanced and build up in places where they shouldn't.

Warming, sweet, and drying, Bai zhu builds up the Spleen Qi, supports the organ in its work, and dries the Dampness that collects when the Spleen is tired. It can help with weak digestion, loose stools, undigested food in the stools, thin mucus congestion in the head and throat (especially when it occurs right after eating), feelings of low energy and lethargy, and bloating and distention. Like Huang qi (astragalus), it can help maintain healthy blood-sugar levels.

<u>Similar herbs:</u> Huang qi (astragalus), Da zao (dates)

PRECAUTIONS: As a Qi tonic it is warming and drying, so be cautious with Heat or insufficient Yin.

Cardamom • Yi zhi ren
Alpiniae oxyphyllae fructus and *Elettaria cardamomum*

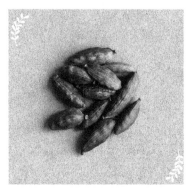

Part used: seeds or whole seed pods

Technically, Yi zhi ren (cardamom) is black cardamom, but I am bending the rules and including green cardamom in this description. Both have similar actions. Green cardamom is true cardamom and the one we think about when we hear the word *cardamom*. It is the flavor found in chai, pumpkin-pie spice blends, and Indian spice blends like korma. It has a sweeter, more palatable flavor than the darker black version. Chinese herbal medicine uses the darker kind, which is spicier and more bitter. Green cardamom is far easier to find, and since it shares so many of the black kind's benefits, for the purposes of this book, it is interchangeable.

Both green and black cardamom are warming and considered Spleen and Kidney Yang tonics. Both help with digestive upset, gas, constipation, and diarrhea. They are especially useful for helping with cold digestion.

Yi zhi ren is anti-inflammatory and antispasmodic and treats constipation, diarrhea, and other stomach problems. Research also shows that cardamom can help with stomach ulcers, colic, and sinus infections, including reducing nasal congestion and sinus headaches.

Similar herbs: Xiao hui xiang (fennel), Rou gui (cinnamon bark), Hu lu ba (fenugreek)

Cat's Claw • Gou teng
Uncariae ramulus cum uncis

Parts used: twigs with hooks

When you see these twigs, you understand why *claw* is in the name. Their job is to anchor Internal Wind, so you can think of the claw as hooking the Wind and pulling it down.

With its coolness, Gou teng (cat's claw) goes to the Liver, Pericardium, and Heart to treat both Internal and External Wind. It is used the most for Internal Wind that is caused by imbalance in the Liver. This is the Wind that comes about when we are lacking fluids to keep the pathways full, which allows Wind to travel through the empty spaces. (Wind is one of the more challenging concepts for a beginner.) Internal Wind causes symptoms in the upper body like eye twitches, headaches, migraines, tremors, or spasms. Gou teng helps with these and with one-sided tinnitus that comes suddenly, feels almost like hearing loss or a loud ringing, then goes away. While it excels at anchoring Internal Wind, it needs to be combined with herbs that treat the underlying cause of insufficient Blood or Yin.

Cook for less than 10 minutes. This herb is a good candidate for infusion, or you may want to add it to your decoction during the last 10 minutes of cooking as part of a formula.

<u>Similar herbs:</u> Bo he (mint), Ju hua (chrysanthemum), Gui zhi (cinnamon twig)

<u>Purchasing:</u> Note that there is a cat's claw of South American origin that is used differently from Chinese Gou teng.

Chrysanthemum • Ju hua
Chrysanthemi morifolii flos

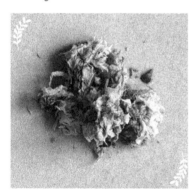

<u>Part used:</u> flowers

Ju hua (chrysanthemum) is in the Release External Wind category. One of its main uses is to support the Lungs and fight colds. Ju hua is sweet, bitter, and slightly cold, so it is particularly helpful for colds that have fevers or sweating; dry, red, itchy eyes; headache; and sore throat. Ju hua is a fabulous herb for the eyes and, with Gou qi zi (goji berry), leads the archetypal formula to help with eye health (Qi Ju Di Huang Wan). It helps the Liver as well, clearing Heat in that system, helping with headaches and facial flushing due to Liver Heat or Liver Fire.

With its cooling properties, Ju hua has been shown by modern research to have anti-inflammatory properties. Research is also showing that unlike traditional usage, Ju hua can help manage type 2 diabetes by regulating blood-sugar levels and fat metabolism.

<u>Similar herbs:</u> Bo he (mint)

PRECAUTIONS: It is slightly cold, so be cautious with long-term use and Spleen Qi deficiency.

Cinnamon Bark • Rou gui
Cinnamomi cassiae cortex

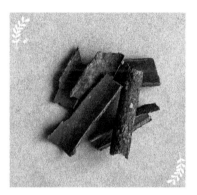

Part used: bark

A far cry from the spice bottle of cinnamon in your pantry, good quality Rou gui (cinnamon bark) is a rich, thick, reddish-brown bark. Going to the Heart, Kidney, Liver, and Spleen, it is acrid, sweet, and warm. It is heating and uplifting and can rescue seriously depleted Yang. It is also a mild diaphoretic and helps with cold damp Bi pain. Other symptoms of Yang deficiency include an aversion to cold, a feeling of cold especially in the back and legs, weakness of the back and legs, infertility, edema, poor appetite, and/or loose stools. There may also be feelings of low energy and lack of motivation.

Research on cinnamon is proving how useful and health-promoting both Rou gui and Gui zhi (cinnamon twig) can be. Much of the research focuses on their ability to help control blood sugar, prediabetes, type 2 diabetes and metabolic syndrome, and high cholesterol. They have also shown promise in helping manage polycystic ovary syndrome (PCOS), a complicated hormone disorder.

Rou gui is not decocted but infused and then added to a decocted formula once it is removed from the heat.

Similar herbs: Hu lu ba (fenugreek), Xiao hui xiang (fennel)

PRECAUTIONS: Due to its warm temperature, be cautious with Yin deficiency and Heat.

Cinnamon Twig • Gui zhi
Cinnamomi cassiae ramulus

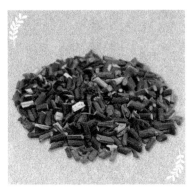

Part used: twigs

A warming herb in the Release External Wind category, Gui zhi (cinnamon twig) is sweet and familiar tasting. It has an archetypal, frequently used formula named after it, Gui Zhi Tang or Cinnamon Twig Decoction. It helps with colds, especially those with cooler symptoms like more chills than fever, no sore throat, or a sore throat that is just scratchy and not sore and painful. Outside of its use for colds and External Wind conditions, Gui zhi helps circulation and mismanaged fluids. It helps formulas for pain, especially when Wind Dampness is present.

Rou gui (cinnamon bark) is the thick, substantial cinnamon bark, but Gui zhi consists of smaller pieces of cinnamon twig that provide different therapeutic benefits. Both are similar in that they are warming and moving. Rou gui is a very warm to hot Yang tonic; Gui zhi is not hot, just warm, and better at treating conditions of Wind. This ability to warm and move stagnation means Gui zhi is included in formulas for that purpose. It warms and unblocks, and warmth and movement also help transform Dampness, making it useful with Bi Dampness that causes pain and stiffness.

Similar herbs: Bo he (mint), Ge gen (kudzu)

PRECAUTIONS: Due to its warm temperature, be cautious with Yin deficiency and Heat.

Cornus Fruit • Shan zhu yu
Corni officinalis fructus

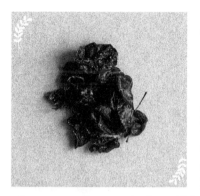

Part used: fruit

This herb is the only one from the Stabilize and Bind category. This action is the opposite of Draining Dampness, as Shan zhu yu (cornus fruit) is astringent; it tones and tightens and prevents the leakage of fluids. When you lose too many fluids, herbs that Stabilize and Bind help rebuild Yin and fluids. Shan zhu yu is sour and slightly warm, helping the Kidney and Liver with excess sweating, dizziness, weakness, and incontinence. It can help normalize a menstrual cycle that continues beyond the average three to six days of bleeding when the excess bleeding is caused by deficiency. It may sound counterintuitive, but a symptom that seems excessive, like too much bleeding or too much sweating, can come from deficiency.

Shan zhu yu benefits the Heart by supporting the Blood and Yin in the Kidney and Liver, which supports the Blood and Yin of the Heart.

During an intake, I always ask my herbal clients whether they sweat and how much. For some, this is an odd question, but it is healthy to sweat when working out or on a hot day, but it isn't healthy to sweat too much or all the time, or at night while you're sleeping when the temperature is moderate. Losing too many fluids can cause you to deplete your Yin and eventually shift your temperature warmer. In Liu Wei Di Huang Wan (Rehmannia Six), the classic formula for building Yin, in addition to herbs that build Yin, Shan zhu yu is included to astringe and preserve fluids.

Menstrual blood can give clues to any underlying patterns. Thin, pale, watery blood is deficient, while darker blood with clots (brown, purple, or very dark red) is more stagnant. Heat shows up in bright red blood.

PRECAUTIONS: Do not use during Exterior Wind invasions (colds and flu) due to its astringent nature.

Cyperus • Xiang fu
Cyperi rotundi rhizoma

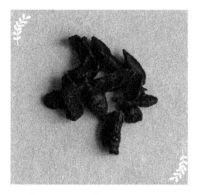

<u>Part used:</u> rhizome

Xiang fu (cyperus) is a strong mover of Qi and is excellent for all sorts of imbalances caused by Qi stagnation, especially pent-up emotions and frustration. Xiang fu, also called nut grass, is inexpensive and easy to grow, so much so that it is listed as a noxious weed in many parts of the United States, with some states listing it as one that needs to be quarantined. When you purchase Xiang fu rhizomes, they are dried and processed and are not viable for growing, so there is no chance of inadvertently spreading this noxious weed that is also a useful herbal medicine.

Commonly used in gynecology for menstrual issues, Xiang fu has an affinity for the Liver and Triple Heater with a neutral temperature. Herbs that affect the Triple Heater are rare. Many Qi movers are warm, and warmth helps movement, so neutral and cool herbs that move the Qi are valuable to know when stagnation has built up Heat. Xiang fu is used along with blood-regulating herbs for injuries and trauma.

While in graduate school, when the workload of classes and clinic made life extra stressful, my classmates and I joked that we should make Xiang fu in sublingual form, so we could instantly soothe our frustration and Liver Qi stagnation.

A human study showed patients taking Xiang fu for three months had a lowering of cholesterol and triglycerides as well as weight loss.

<u>Similar herbs:</u> Chen pi (tangerine peel)

Dates (Jujube) • Da zao
Zizyphi jujubae fructus

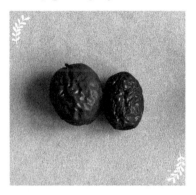

Part used: fruit

Sweet, warm, and nourishing for the Earth element, Da zao (dates) helps build the Qi and Blood of the Spleen and Stomach. Da zao can build up Qi without being drying or draining fluids and can calm the Shen in the Heart through building the Qi and Blood that support it. As you age, Yin deficiency becomes a more common pattern. Aging is the process of getting drier. We are gooey and full of Yin and fluids when we are born but slowly lose the fullness of Yin. Menopausal symptoms come from Yin-deficient Heat. After middle age, it can be a challenge to tonify Spleen Qi without being overly drying or warming to the Yin. Da zao can help with that balance.

Da zao is one of the trio of herbs affectionately known as the "three sweets." They are Da zao, Sheng jiang (ginger), and Zhi gan cao (honey-fried licorice). With so many bitter herbs and flavors, Chinese formulas almost always have one to three of the three sweets to help with digestion and to balance flavor. As Mary Poppins would say, they are the spoonful of sugar to make the medicine go down.

Similar herbs: Bai zhu (atractylodes), Huang qi (astragalus)

Purchasing: Hong zao are specifically red dates and are interchangeable with Da zao. Both Hong zao and Da zao differ from dates (like Medjool) that come from the date palm tree.

Fennel • Xiao hui xiang
Foeniculi vulgaris fructus

Part used: seed

Warm and acrid, Xiao hui xiang (fennel) helps move and warm. Cold temperature slows movement, like water that freezes into ice, and the result is stillness. Cold can cause stagnation and pain. While this can come from very cold weather or cold food, it can also come from being in contact with something cold. An example is that of athletes competing, being warm, and then sitting on cold benches. The cold enters meridians like the Liver channel that come into contact with the cold bench—an example of an External cause of disease.

By warming and moving and going to the Spleen, Stomach, Liver, and Kidney channels, Xiao hui xiang soothes abdominal cramping as well as uterine cramping and pain. It can also work quickly if the condition has just begun. I had a friend in Michigan who—in the middle of a cold winter—was eating cold foods like yogurt for breakfast and lunch. He started having painful cramps in his stomach that even radiated to his sides and back at times. A formula of warm herbs like Xiao hui xiang stopped the pain the same day, and with a shift to warmer-temperature foods, the pain did not return.

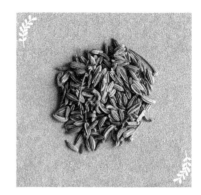

Similar herbs: Hu lu ba (fenugreek)

Fenugreek • Hu lu ba
Trigonellae foeni-graeci semen

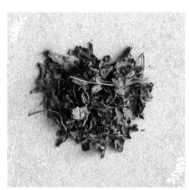

Part used: seed

A warming Kidney Yang tonic that treats Cold in the Lower Jiao or lower abdomen with feelings of heaviness, aversion to cold, and pain (including a sore, weak lower back and knees). Kidney Yang deficiency can also show up as sexual imbalances like impotence and infertility, lack of motivation to start new projects, poor appetite, loose stools, edema in the legs, and abundant clear urination. A lack of sufficient Kidney Yang means no organ system in the body has enough, and it can look like exhaustion.

There is significant research to support using Hu lu ba (fenugreek) to help manage blood sugar, insulin resistance, type 2 diabetes, weight loss, and high cholesterol. Some studies even show its promise in slowing the growth of some cancers.

Similar herbs: Rou gui (cinnamon bark), Xu duan (teasel)

PRECAUTIONS: If prediabetic or diabetic, you'll need to monitor blood sugar.

Goji Berry • Gou qi zi
Lycii chinensis fructus

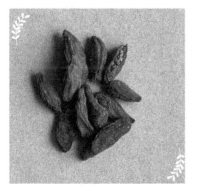

<u>Part used:</u> fruit

The goji berry's rich red color hints at its gift for building Blood. It is nutritive and nourishing. Sometimes called wolfberry, it is one of the premiere herbs for eye health in the Chinese *Materia Medica*. Gou qi zi (goji berry) helps nourish the Liver, Lung, and Kidney systems. Some sources even say that Gou qi zi builds the Kidney Yang as well as the Yin.

Gou qi zi has gained increasing recognition over the last decade, but it's been part of the Chinese herbalist's dispensary for much longer. Gou qi zi is the red berry of the *Lycium* plant. With its sweet and tangy flavor, it can be eaten fresh or dried, but finding it fresh in the United States is challenging. It is far easier to find it in its dried form, which can be enjoyed like other dried berries and fruits. The dried berries can be used in snack and trail mixes, or you can soak them and use them in smoothies or cooking. In Chinese diagnostic terms, goji berry builds the Blood and Yin of the Liver and Kidney and is an overall nutritive tonic. It is recommended for people who have low energy, anemia, trouble falling (or staying) asleep, and lower back pain. It is one of the best herbs in Chinese herbal medicine for eye health.

Di gu pi (lycium bark) is the bark of the lycium tree; it is cold and sweet, cools the Blood, and works to clear Heat in the Lungs and Kidney.

<u>Similar herbs:</u> Sang shen (mulberry), Long yan rou (longan berry)

<u>Growing:</u> The goji plant can be cultivated in many areas of the United States. It is not a fussy plant and can thrive where other fruits might struggle, like in the dry, arid climate of the Mountain West. Di gu pi is the bark of the goji plant.

Hawthorn • Shan zha
Crataegi fructus

Part used: berry

Hawthorn is a common supplement and much loved by Western herbalists. However, Western and Chinese herbalists use hawthorn in very different ways. Western and Chinese hawthorn are different varieties, although the trees and fruits can look similar, and Chinese hawthorn is not used for cardiovascular and heart health. Chinese Shan zha (hawthorn) is categorized as an herb for Food Stagnation and could be compared to a digestive enzyme. It would be used when digestion is slow or for overeating in a post-Thanksgiving formula.

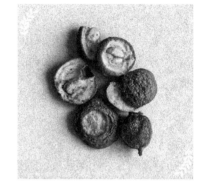

Western herbalists use Shan zha as a cardiotonic herb that has research supporting its use in many cardiovascular diseases. However, in Chinese medicine its main role is to alleviate food stagnation.

Note: This is the only herb in the Food Stagnation category.

Job's Tears • Yi yi ren
Coicis lachryma-jobi semen

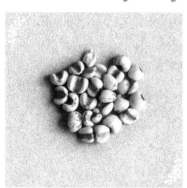

Part used: seed

Yi yi ren (Job's tears) is all about draining Dampness from the three organ systems that help control and store water: the Lung, Spleen, and Kidney. Yi yi ren indirectly boosts the Qi of these systems by taking some of the workload from them. It is used for conditions of excess fluid like edema and excess vaginal discharge.

Dampness can also cause pain. Joint pain caused by Dampness is called Bi. Yi yi ren is used to treat Bi-syndrome pain and is combined with other herbs to address all the patterns behind the pain. It has also been found to decrease blood glucose and insulin levels, with research proving this antidiabetic action.

Similar herbs: Fu ling (poria), Du huo (angelica)

Kudzu • Ge gen
Puerariae radix

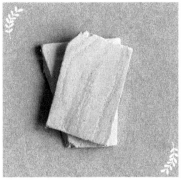

Part used: root

Yes, this is the same kudzu that has been trying to take over the southern United States. However, much of the supply found in US herbal apothecaries still comes from China. I have heard firsthand accounts of how challenging kudzu root can be to wild harvest, but a good solution to the invasive growth of kudzu in the South could be to harvest it for use by Chinese herbalists in the United States.

Ge gen (kudzu) is sweet and acrid, with a cool temperature that is traditionally found in the Release External Wind category. It is found in formulas to help with colds and to relax tense muscles, especially the neck and shoulders. It has moistening properties, helping when there is a fever and thirst with a cold.

To put Ge gen in a single category is to ignore many other wonderful things about the plant. It can clear rashes and has an uplifting energetic. There are multiple areas of study with Ge gen right now, including preventing age-related macular degeneration and improving eye health. Ge gen has proven in scientific studies to lower alcohol consumption: When given a chance to drink, participants in these studies consumed alcohol more slowly and did less binge drinking.

Similar herbs: Bo he (mint), Ju hua (chrysanthemum), Gou teng (cat's claw)

Ligusticum • Chuan xiong
Ligustici chuanxiong rhizoma

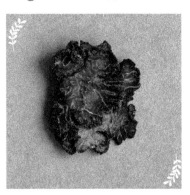

Part used: root

Warm, acrid Chuan xiong (ligusticum) is in the Regulate Blood category. In Chinese medicine the term *regulate* is used, because the goal is to have the Blood, including its circulation and consistency, in balance. *Regulate* denotes restoring the movement to healthy levels, and that can include herbs that help stop bleeding or do the opposite of moving blood. As with other herbs that Regulate Blood, Chuan xiong is useful in menstrual disorders where pain and clots are present.

Chuan xiong has an affinity for the upper body and head and is used in combination with other herbs for headaches with different underlying patterns. By itself, it is a useful addition to cold formulas in which the cold is accompanied by a headache. It is also used in topical formulas for trauma and injuries.

Another common name for Chuan xiong is Szechuan lovage.

<u>Similar herbs:</u> Jiang huang (turmeric), Dan shen (salvia)

Longan Berry • Long yan rou
Euphoriae longanae arillus

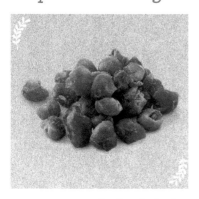

<u>Part used:</u> fruit

A fruit that can be found fresh in Asian groceries when it is in season, Long yan rou (longan berry) helps the Liver and Spleen, building Blood and calming the Shen. Delicious enough to be eaten alone, it can be purchased dried year-round. Long yan rou helps with trouble sleeping, palpitations, and memory lapses. Long yan rou supports the Earth element when you have been working and thinking too much. The Spleen helps you recall information, and when you are overworked and tired, you can experience problems with memory and retrieval of information.

Many of the herbs in this chapter are divided into Qi and Blood tonics, doing one or the other but working together. Like the herbs that build and support them, Qi and Blood work together and support each other, with sufficient Qi needed to make Blood. Long yan rou is a bridge between Qi and Blood tonics, being a Liver and Heart Blood tonic while also going to the Spleen, which is in charge of the Qi. Long-term use of Long yan rou is said to prevent aging and nourish the spirit.

<u>Similar herbs:</u> Gou qi zi (goji berry), Sang shen (mulberry)

<u>Growing:</u> Longan trees can grow in the warmest zones of the United States, like southern Florida.

Mint • Bo he
Menthae haplocalycis herba

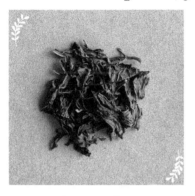

Parts used: aerial parts, leaves

While not exactly the same as the mint you buy at the grocery store or garden center, this is very similar. Mint is an inexpensive, easy-to-grow herb, so it's not difficult to find sustainable sources.

Bo he (mint) is in the category Cool, Acrid Release External Wind, meaning one of its uses is to help the Lung energy and fight off colds. A cold that calls for Bo he could have associated fever and chills, sweating, a sore or scratchy throat, and dry, itchy eyes.

As an herb for the Lung and Liver systems, it also helps with red, hot skin conditions like rashes. It can also help gently move hot, stagnant Liver Qi and the pain or emotions associated with stuck Qi.

Bo he should be infused, not decocted. When drinking it alone, infuse; when adding it to a formula with other herbs that are cooked longer, add during the last few minutes of cooking.

Similar herbs: Ju hua (chrysanthemum)

Note: While Bo he is a specific kind of mint, most mints and peppermints can be used interchangeably.

Mulberry • Sang shen
Mori albae fructus

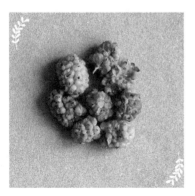

Part used: fruit

I have included Sang shen (mulberry) partly because it is a delicious part of the Chinese herbal *Materia Medica* but also because throughout neighborhoods there are helpful mulberry trees being ignored or complained about when the berries fall and make a mess. By learning to harvest these nutritious purple fruits, you can help prevent the mess made by uncollected fruits while gathering a useful Blood tonic. They can also be purchased dried.

Sang shen is a sweet-flavored Blood tonic that supports the Liver Blood. Symptoms of Blood deficiency include floaters (small dark shapes in the visual field), scanty periods, paleness, and tendency to feel cold. Research shows that mulberries are hepatoprotective (liver protective) and balance cholesterol and that they help with obesity, liver disease, diabetes, cardiovascular diseases, and cancer.

<u>Similar herbs:</u> Gou qi zi (goji berry), Bai shao (peony)

<u>Purchasing:</u> Sang shen zi is found in the category of Expel Wind Dampness and is the twig of the mulberry tree.

Ophiopogon • Mai men dong
Ophiopogonis japonici tuber

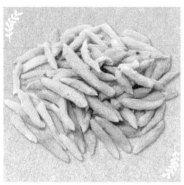

<u>Part used:</u> root

A cooling Yin tonic for the Stomach, Lung, and Heart, Mai men dong (ophiopogon) cools and nourishes the Lungs and helps maintain proper moisture levels in the body. When you don't have enough Stomach Yin, you experience digestive upset like heartburn or excessive hunger and imbalanced digestion. Mai men dong (ophiopogon) soothes the heat and rebuilds the Yin. It also helps with dry constipation.

Yin also keeps the Lungs healthy with the appropriate level of fluids: not too wet, not too dry. Dryness causes coughs, wheezing, pain, and constriction in the chest. Modern research shows benefits with the use of Mai men dong for mild to moderate asthma.

The third system this herb helps is the Yin of the Heart. Remember the story of the Shen (page 10), the spirit that resides in the Heart? The Shen needs a soft, comfortable place to rest for us to be fully present and centered. Mai men dong helps make this soft space for the Shen, helping with emotional upset, insomnia with vivid dreams, and irritability.

<u>Similar herbs:</u> Tian men dong (asparagus root)

PRECAUTIONS: Yin tonics are often dense, thick materials that can be hard to digest, so combine with herbs to help with Spleen Qi deficiency and digestion when needed.

Peony (White) • Bai shao
Paeoniae radix alba

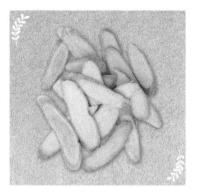

Part used: root

Many Chinese herbal medicines include the name *peony*, such as red peony, tree peony, and Bai shao, the white peony root. A Blood and Yin tonic for the Liver and Spleen systems, Bai shao (peony) excels at nourishing the ligaments, tendons, and muscles to ensure healthy, smooth movement. It is an often-used herb in musculoskeletal formulas.

Cool, bitter, and sour, Bai shao helps with the symptoms of Liver Blood and Yin deficiency, like trouble falling asleep or staying asleep, night sweats, and floaters in the vision. Another sign of Blood deficiency is having cold fingers and toes; this is because you may not have enough Blood to supply the entire body, so the fingers and toes get left out of the warming circulation. Sometimes when you start to run low on Blood and Yin, you can start to get warmer, so the coolness of Bai shao is welcome to balance temperature.

In Chinese herbal medicine, herbs can have a mental and emotional benefit as well. Bai shao helps with low self-esteem and lack of fluidity and smoothness with emotions. The Liver is known as the General, who leads us forward according to the larger vision and plan. Bai shao makes sure the General isn't too rigid with the plan and can adapt to fluctuations or changes in the plan. Bai shao is found in formulas developed by martial artists, because of its helpful actions on the musculoskeletal system but also for its role in supporting and maintaining flexibility.

Similar herbs: Gou qi zi (goji berry) and Sang shen (mulberry)

Purchasing: With multiple peony products available, make sure you are buying Bai shao (white peony).

Poria • Fu ling
Poriae cocos sclerotium

Part used: the whole mushroom

Fu ling (poria) is a sweet, bland herb with a neutral temperature that drains Dampness and supports the Heart, Spleen, Kidney, and Lung systems. It is often paired with Spleen Qi building herbs like Bai zhu (atractylodes), so that as the Spleen Qi tonic strengthens the Spleen, the Dampness that the Spleen was too tired to manage is also taken care of, helping lighten its workload.

Dampness and Phlegm can cause problems and make any existing imbalances worse. Fu ling is common in formulas due to the importance of draining excess fluid. Because of its affinity for the Heart and its sweetness, it can quiet the Heart and calm the spirit.

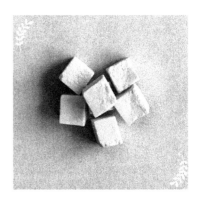

Similar herbs: Yi yi ren (Job's tears)

PRECAUTIONS: Because Fu ling is drying, use it in formulation if Yin deficiency is present.

Note: Poria is also known as Hoelen or Tuckahoe.

Reishi Mushroom • Ling zhi
Ganoderma lucidum

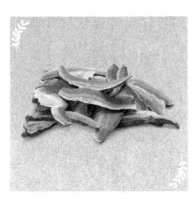

Part used: fruiting mushroom

Mushrooms are so popular, these days you can buy blends of mushrooms and even mushroom coffee substitutes. Ling zhi (reishi) is a tonic for the Qi and Blood of the Heart, Liver, and Lungs. A highly valued herb throughout history, it calms the Shen and assists emotional health by supporting Qi and Blood in the Heart. As it builds the Lung Qi, it helps with coughing, wheezing, and shortness of breath. Its overall tonic properties strengthen digestion and help alleviate dryness and a tendency toward cold hands and feet.

Ling zhi has antiaging effects: It balances blood sugar while strengthening the heart and cardiovascular system. It also helps with memory. Research also shows antineuro-degeneration, antioxidant, antitumor, liver-protective, and immunomodulatory capabilities.

Similar herbs: Da zao (dates), Gou qi zi (goji berry), He huan pi and He huan hua (albizzia)

PRECAUTIONS: Buy from a reputable source so that you know the mushroom has been properly identified; monitor blood sugar if prediabetic or diabetic.

Rosebud • Mei gui hua
Rosae rugosae flos

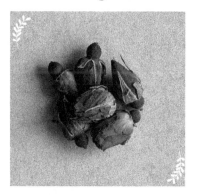

Part used: rosebud

At some point, everyone should open a container of Mei gui hua (rosebud), hold their face close, and inhale. The small, closed buds of *Rosa rugosa* are pink, with a sweet taste and delightful aroma.

Mei gui hua has a sweet flavor and moves stagnant Liver Qi in a gentle but effective way. It helps with irregular periods, especially with cycles that are shorter than the standard 28 to 32 days. Any pain before or during the first day of a menstrual cycle is indicative of Qi stagnation, as are some standard PMS symptoms such as irritability and frustration.

Mei gui hua is proof that to be effective, an herb doesn't have to work like a sledgehammer. Despite appearing delicate, it can be used as a topical for trauma and pain as well. In Western herbalism, Mei gui hua goes to the heart and is used to calm and cool the heart and emotions.

<u>Similar herbs:</u> Xiang fu (cyperus), He huan pi and He huan hua (albizzia)

<u>Purchasing:</u> Look for closed buds, not loose petals.

Salvia • Dan shen
Salviae miltiorrhizae radix

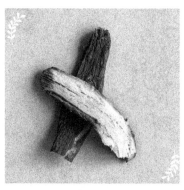

Part used: root

Bitter and cold, Dan shen (salvia) treats Heat and Blood stagnation in the Heart and Liver with symptoms like insomnia with dream-disturbed sleep, restlessness, irritability, and palpitations. Heat rises and is upsetting and unsettling for the Heart and the Shen and often shows through emotions as well, making them more emphatic and possibly more unpredictable or erratic. Dan shen is also known as mildly Blood-building.

Dan shen is a Blood mover and as such is often used for gynecological conditions where Blood stagnation is causing menstrual irregularities like pain, clotting, and irregular cycles. Blood stagnation causes pain that is sharp and stabbing in a fixed location. Trauma, injuries, and bruises are examples of Blood stagnation from external causes, with internal Blood stagnation showing up in cardiovascular and menstrual conditions. Internal Blood stagnation in people with periods will show up as menstrual pain and clots in the menstrual blood for the entire period. (Small clots on just the first day of menstruation could be Qi stagnation.) Dan shen can also be used topically for Blood stagnation due to injuries and trauma.

Another common name for Dan shen is red sage root.

<u>Similar herbs:</u> Chuan xiong (ligusticum), Jiang huang (turmeric)

PRECAUTIONS: Do not use herbs that treat Blood stagnation concurrently with blood thinners, during pregnancy, or while nursing. Use caution and monitor with other cardiovascular medications.

Tangerine Peel • Chen pi
Citri reticulatae pericarpium

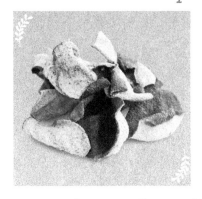

<u>Part used:</u> ripe outer peel of the fruit

Citrus peels are used in Chinese herbal medicine. Chen pi (tangerine peel) is the ripe peel of the tangerine. Chen pi moves the Qi in the Spleen and Stomach. If you use the unripe, green tangerine peel, it is called Qing pi, and it has a much stronger moving action. The gentler, mature Chen pi is used in formulas to balance herbs that build Qi. It's like making pasta and dumping the pasta into boiling water. Often, the pasta can clump and stick together, so you need to stir it. Chen pi is like the spoon stirring all the building, nourishing herbs so that they don't stick and clump together but instead "cook" evenly for optimal energy and optimal absorption of nutrition.

Stuck Qi will show itself through pain and distention; it can also show up as emotional stuckness and pain. Moving and circulating Qi smoothly takes Qi, so Qi movers and Qi builders are often used together. Chen pi also dries Dampness and helps with digestive upset, including belching and slow digestion. It has been shown in studies to be a useful ally in patients with cancer by having antitumor and anticarcinogenic effects.

<u>Similar herbs:</u> Xiang fu (cyperus)

Teasel • Xu duan
Dipsaci radix

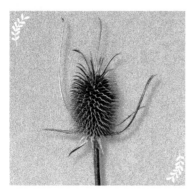

Part used: root

Xu duan (teasel) is a warming tonic for the Kidneys, building up Yang when you run low. Yang is the bright, warm force that lifts and dries and keeps you moving. Yang tonic herbs support the structure of your body to keep you upright and moving, strengthening your lower back, knees, legs, and ankles.

Feeling cold and lethargic or heavy, having low libido or an achy and weak back, or hitting snooze a few times plus needing coffee just to wake up after a good night's sleep can all indicate deficient Yang.

Pain in the back and lower limbs that responds well to warmth like a heating pad, massage, and pressure is indicative of a Yang deficiency and calls for Xu duan. This kind of pain may not improve with movement, especially significant amounts of exercise, because it could further deplete Yang.

Similar herbs: Rou gui (cinnamon bark), Hu lu ba (fenugreek)

PRECAUTIONS: Use with care if Heat and Yang excess are present.

Tree Peony • Mu dan pi
Paeoniae moutan cortex

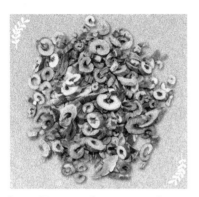

Part used: bark

There are two kinds of Heat: full (or excess) and deficient (or empty). In the category of Clear Heat, Mu dan pi (tree peony) is cooling, bitter, and acrid. It is used to clear Heat, including the empty Heat that builds up with Yin deficiency, when the cooling Yin is running low and Heat starts to build. One analogy about Yin is that it is like the water in a radiator, keeping the engine cool. If the water runs low, the engine can start to run warm and eventually overheat. This overheating is often seen in menopause with sweating and night sweats, hot flashes, dryness, and symptoms worse at night. Heat likes to rise, so Mu dan pi is helpful for signs of Heat in the head, like dry, red eyes, headache, and malar flush, in which just the cheeks get red and warm. In more extreme cases, there can be "steaming bone disorder," in which you have the sensation of your bones feeling hot. I've seen a few menopausal women with this, and it is very uncomfortable. For treating Heat caused by deficiency, Mu dan pi works well with Blood and Yin tonics like Gou qi zi (goji berry), Bai shao (peony), and Tian men dong (asparagus root). For full Heat, it can be combined with other cold or cooling herbs.

Bleeding excessively during menstruation has many underlying patterns; Mu dan pi helps with the kind of bleeding that comes from excess Heat.

Similar herbs: Ju hua (chrysanthemum), Bo he (mint)

Tricosanthes • Gua lou
Tricosanthis kirlowii fructus

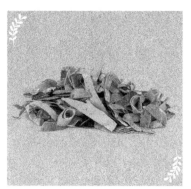

<u>Part used:</u> the whole gourd

Found in the category of Transform Phlegm, Stop Coughing, Gua lou (tricosanthes) is cold and helps with hot or feverish conditions that include a cough with phlegm that might be getting thicker, stickier, and harder to expectorate. It helps the Lungs and their paired organ, the Large Intestine, as well as the Stomach.

Seeds are available at Strictly Medicinal, and you can grow this gourd in your garden. When you buy Gua lou, it is recognizable as a dried slice of a gourd with seeds inside. The seeds can be used alone and are known as Gua lou ren (tricosanthes seed).

<u>Similar herbs:</u> Zi wan (aster)

PRECAUTIONS: Do not use during pregnancy without the supervision of a licensed practitioner.

<u>Note:</u> Another common name for this is Chinese snake gourd.

Turmeric • Jiang huang
Curcumae longae rhizoma

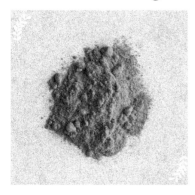

<u>Part used:</u> rhizome

Jiang huang (turmeric) moves Blood that has become stagnant. (Remember that the Chinese concept of Blood does not always correlate exactly to the Western definition of blood.) Blood stagnation causes pain that is sharp and stabbing in a fixed location. Trauma, injuries, and bruises are examples of Blood stagnation from external causes. Internal Blood stagnation is seen in cardiovascular conditions, and in people with periods it will show up as menstrual pain and clots during their cycle. Jiang huang is also used in topicals for trauma and injuries, including Bi-syndrome pain, which involves Dampness.

<u>Similar herbs:</u> Chuan xiong (ligusticum), Dan shen (salvia)

PRECAUTIONS: Dosages used in cooking are generally regarded as safe. Do not use herbs that treat Blood stagnation concurrently with blood thinners.

<u>Growing:</u> If you live in a warm climate or have a greenhouse, you can grow your own Jiang huang.

<u>Purchasing:</u> You can find it fresh in grocery stores. When buying the herb powdered, get it from a reputable source to guarantee its quality.

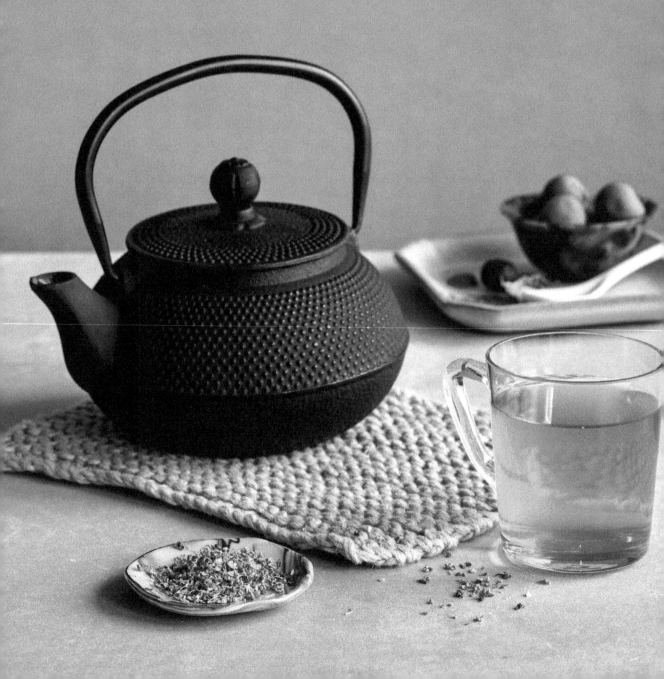

Infusion for
Falling Asleep, PAGE 143

Part Three

FORMULAS
AND REMEDIES

Here, you'll find a simplified, shortened version of a Chinese herbal formulas and strategies textbook. This final section takes all you have learned in the three previous chapters and puts it into action. It combines single herbs into remedies or formulas and explains how each combination of herbs works in terms of Chinese medicine.

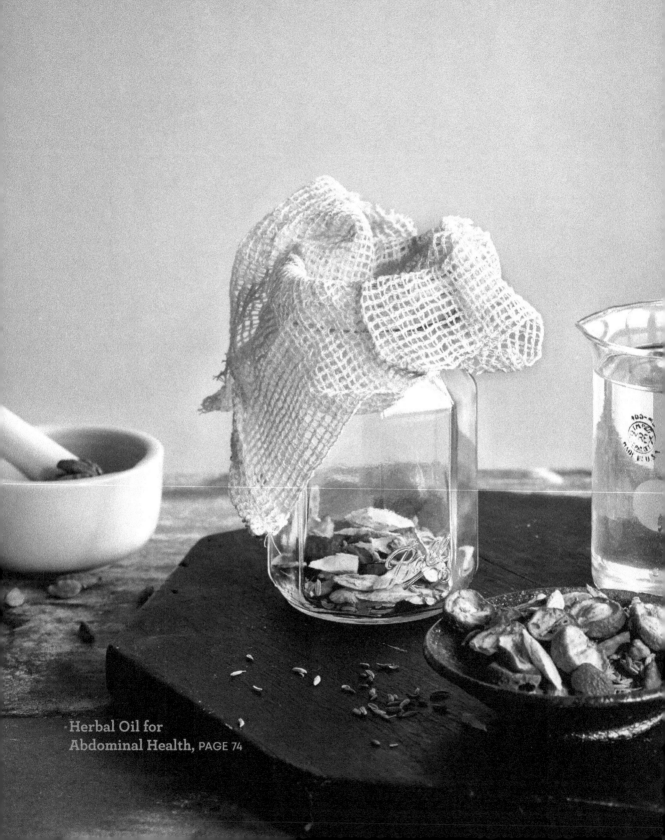

Herbal Oil for
Abdominal Health, PAGE 74

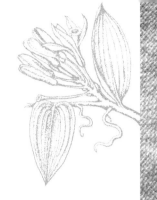

CHAPTER 4

Formulas and Remedies

In this chapter are 110 formulas or remedies for various conditions. Chinese herbal formulas often have longer, more complicated lists of ingredients that easily number as many as 12 to 18 different herbs! For the purposes of this book, the formulas are simplified with fewer ingredients, to make them safe and accessible for the beginner.

The formulas are organized by ailment and how they help balance the body. In a traditional collection of Chinese formulas, they would be divided by category (e.g., Tonify Yin or Regulate Blood). For each formula, I attempt to stay true to Chinese formulas and explain how the herbs work together and the patterns that they treat.

I recommend that you keep track of the remedies you try and why. It's so easy to forget how you felt four weeks—or four months—before you started with herbs, and improvements can go unnoticed unless you take the time to remember and compare. As a practitioner, every few weeks or months I check in with my patients about symptoms or imbalances they were concerned with, reminding them of how they rated their concern or discomfort in the beginning and asking how they would rate it after their herbal protocol. Sometimes, a condition can improve or resolve, and people don't realize it until they are asked. It may seem odd, but many times I've heard patients express surprise that something is better, and as it gradually improved, the improvement became the new normal.

Taking notes in a journal or a planner or calendar can be helpful—for example, "Feeling low energy with digestive upset and starting this herbal remedy." Then, make a note or schedule a check-in several weeks out to see how your energy level and digestion compare after your herbal regimen. As a practitioner, I create custom formulas for my patients that they usually take for months; every month or so I adjust the formula as their situation evolves.

THE IMPORTANCE OF PATTERNS

One rule I repeat often is "treat excesses before—or while—you treat deficiencies." If someone has excesses, such as Dampness, Qi stagnation, or Heat or Blood stagnation, and they take only tonics, because they also have signs of deficiency, they will most likely feel worse. That leads to my *other* most repeated phrase: "Find the patterns and treat the patterns." As you proceed, know that tonics that build you up are lovely, but if you are stuck or hot or damp, moving or clearing that blockage can free up the energy you do have and help you feel better.

About the Formulas

Cooking Chinese herbal medicines isn't an exact science. Herbs are processed into different sizes—sometimes even with the same supplier. All herbs are dried unless otherwise noted, as that is how most Chinese herbs are supplied and sold. Due to the variations that occur naturally, all liquid amounts will vary depending on how much water the dried herbs absorb. During preparation, always feel free to add more water if needed.

To be user-friendly, the ingredients in smaller formulas are measured in teaspoons and tablespoons. However, with larger amounts (e.g., formulas for a full week), grams are listed to ensure correct amounts.

Single Herb Sampling

MAKES 1 CUP

Any of the 35 herbs listed in our *Materia Medica* can be tried alone. When I teach Chinese herbal medicine classes, I enjoy having "sampling" herbs and formulas for my students to try. It not only gives them an idea of the flavors and tastes they are asking others to ingest, but it also lets them experience how—and where—you feel the formulas in your body. Is it warm, and does it make your stomach feel good? Do you feel relaxed and calm or energized? Follow the instructions on how to prepare each herb and explore by sampling for yourself.

1 to 2 teaspoons of a single herb

1½ cups water

Most of the herbs in these formulas can be decocted, but Mei gui hua (rosebud), He huan hua (albizzia flower), and Rou gui (cinnamon bark) are prepared via infusion only. Chen pi (tangerine peel), Bo he (mint), and Gui zhi (cinnamon twig) are limited to 10 minutes of decoction time. The rest can be decocted for much longer times, preferably at least 20 minutes.

TO MAKE A DECOCTION:

1. Place the herbs in a non-aluminum saucepan and add the water.
2. Bring the mixture to a boil, then simmer uncovered for 20 minutes.
3. Strain and drink while warm. Take a few quiet moments while sipping to really experience the decoction.
4. Drink the same day. Chinese herbal formulas should be taken warm, not cold, so add more hot water if the drink cools.

1. Place the herbs in a teapot, large mug, or coffee press. Boil the water and pour it over the herbs.

2. Infuse, covered, for at least an hour. For a stronger infusion, steep longer or even overnight.

3. Strain and drink while warm. Take a few quiet moments while sipping to really experience the infusion.

4. Drink the same day. Chinese herbal formulas should be taken warm, not cold, so add more hot water if the drink cools.

Abdominal Pain

The abdomen can be a source of aches and unease, nausea, and minor digestive upset. Herbs can help ease cramping and pain and improve digestion to prevent further discomfort.

Herbal Oil for Abdominal Health

MAKES ONE 16-OUNCE PINT JAR

Many traditional healing systems use the navel (at the center of your body). In qigong and tai chi, the navel is the focal point of exercises to support Stomach and Spleen Qi. This belly oil can be used with qigong belly circles: Imagine a clock on your stomach, with the center of the clock at the belly button. Gently rub the oil in a clockwise direction, like you are following the numbers on the edge of the clock. Only light pressure should be used, and the pace should be slow and calming. For babies and children, rubbing belly circles can help with all sorts of abdominal pains. It makes an excellent addition to bedtime routines.

12 to 15 Yi zhi ren (cardamom) pods, crushed

5 pieces Da zao (dates), chopped

10 to 12 pieces Shan zha (hawthorn)

¼ cup Huang qi (astragalus)

3 teaspoons Xiao hui xiang (fennel)

About 14 ounces oil of your choice

1. Fill a 16-ounce glass container with the Yi zhi ren, Da zao, Shan zha, Huang qi, and Xiao hui xiang, leaving space between the top of the herbs and the top of the jar.

2. Cover the herbs completely with the oil and secure the lid. (It is important that no herbs are above the oil and remain uncovered, as this can ruin the oil.)

3. Let the oil sit for 6 weeks, then strain and store in a glass container. Store in the refrigerator and use within 6 months to a year.

4. Use 1 to 3 tablespoons for abdominal massage. This oil can be gently warmed before applying.

Aches and Pains

Bi (pronounced "bee") pain is a combination of Wind and Dampness causing pain and achiness that get worse with weather or humidity. It is not sharp or stabbing; it can move around; and it can be hard to pinpoint the precise spot where it hurts. Bi pain starts as cold in temperature and can stay cold or heat up over time due to any stagnation or environmental factor like humidity, heat, or cold.

Decoction for Aches and Pains

MAKES 7 CUPS

This decoction focuses on Bi pain that is cold. Often, Bi pain occurs along with Yang deficiency and includes symptoms like feeling cold, a weak lower back and legs, and low energy or fatigue.

15 grams Du huo (angelica)

12 grams Yi yi ren (Job's tears)

9 grams Jiang huang (turmeric)

9 grams Xu duan (teasel)

8 cups water

9 grams Gui zhi (cinnamon twig)

6 grams Rou gui (cinnamon bark)

1. Place the Du huo, Yi yi ren, Jiang huang, and Xu duan in a non-aluminum saucepan and add the water.

2. Bring the mixture to a boil, then simmer uncovered for 25 minutes.

3. Add the Gui zhi and simmer for another 5 minutes. Remove from the heat.

4. Strain into a large, 8-cup glass measuring cup. If the total amount is less than 7 cups, add water to bring the mixture to 7 cups total.

5. Add the Rou gui to the strained decoction and infuse, covered, for at least one hour. The Rou gui pieces can stay in the decoction even after you refrigerate for further infusion and strength.

6. Set aside ½ cup as the first dose to drink immediately, then refrigerate the rest.

7. Drink ½ cup morning and evening for 1 week. After 7 days, discard any remaining decoction and make a new batch.

Decoction for Aches and Pains with Heat

MAKES 7 CUPS

This formula is similar to the other formula for Bi pain, but the ingredients shift so it can deal better with the Heat that has built up. Along with the warm ingredients that move and drain the Dampness and stagnation, Mu dan pi (tree peony) and Bai shao (peony) are added to cool the Heat that has developed.

15 grams Du huo (angelica)

12 grams Yi yi ren (Job's tears)

12 grams Mu dan pi (tree peony)

9 grams Jiang huang (turmeric)

9 grams Bai shao (peony)

8 cups water

9 grams Gui zhi (cinnamon twig)

1. Place the Du huo, Yi yi ren, Mu dan pi, Jiang huang, and Bai shao in a non-aluminum saucepan and add the water.

2. Bring the mixture to a boil, then simmer uncovered for 25 minutes.

3. Add the Gui zhi and simmer for another 5 minutes. Remove from the heat.

4. Strain into a large, 8-cup glass measuring cup. If the total amount is less than 7 cups, add water to bring the mixture to 7 cups total.

5. Set aside ½ cup as the first dose to drink immediately, then refrigerate the rest.

6. Drink ½ cup morning and evening for 1 week. After 7 days, discard any remaining decoction and make a new batch.

Compress for Aches and Pains

MAKES ENOUGH FOR 5 DAYS

For achy pain that is colder and feels better with heat, this formula includes warming ingredients. Wrapping the compress in another cloth can help preserve its warmth.

½ cup Du huo (angelica)

½ cup Yi yi ren (Job's tears)

¼ cup Rou gui (cinnamon bark)

¼ cup Xiao hui xiang (fennel)

8 cups water

½ cup Gui zhi (cinnamon twig)

Clean, dry cloth

1. Place the Du huo, Yi yi ren, Rou gui, and Xiao hui xiang in a non-aluminum saucepan and add the water.

2. Bring the mixture to a boil, then simmer uncovered for 25 minutes.

3. Add the Gui zhi and simmer for another 5 minutes. Remove from the heat.

4. Strain into a large, 8-cup glass measuring cup.

5. Wash the area to be soaked, soak the cloth in the warm herbal decoction, and apply to the area for 15 to 30 minutes.

6. Store the decoction in the refrigerator and use it again for up to 5 days. To warm the decoction before using the compress on subsequent days, you can add boiling water or microwave the decoction. You want the compress to be warm to very warm; test the temperature to ensure it is not too hot and will not burn the skin.

Compress for Aches and Pains with Heat

MAKES ENOUGH FOR 5 DAYS

For achy pain that does not like heat or if there is redness, this formula has cooler ingredients. Wrapping the compress in another cloth can help preserve its warmth.

½ cup Du huo (angelica)

½ cup Ge gen (kudzu)

¼ cup Dan shen (salvia) or
　　Mu dan pi (tree peony)

¼ cup Yi yi ren (Job's tears)

8 cups water

½ cup Gui zhi
　　(cinnamon twig)

Clean, dry cloth

1. Place the Du huo, Ge gen, Dan shen (or Mu dan pi), and Yi yi ren in a non-aluminum saucepan and add the water.

2. Bring the mixture to a boil, then simmer uncovered for 25 minutes.

3. Add the Gui zhi and simmer for another 5 minutes. Remove from the heat.

4. Strain into a large, 8-cup glass measuring cup.

5. Wash the area to be soaked, soak the cloth in the warm herbal decoction, and apply to the area for 15 to 30 minutes.

6. Store the decoction in the refrigerator and use it again for up to 5 days. To warm the decoction before using the compress on subsequent days, you can add boiling water or microwave the decoction. You want the compress to be warm to very warm; test the temperature to ensure it is not too hot and will not burn the skin.

PRECAUTIONS: Do not use Dan shen (salvia) with prescription blood thinners; substitute Mu dan pi (tree peony).

Allergies

Allergies can have a similar presentation to colds, and from the Chinese herbal point of view both can be an External Wind invasion. The formulas for cold and allergies are similar as well, but a key with allergies is to start taking the formula before they flare up.

Decoction for Allergies

MAKES 7 CUPS

This formula can help with allergies, but it works best as a preventive. Starting this formula a month before you would usually get seasonal allergies can help build the Lung Qi, which is responsible for the Wei Qi that helps protect us like a shield and can be seen as part of the immune system. This formula, or others that build Qi, can be used before cold season in a similar way to build immunity. This remedy is best taken for a few weeks to a few months; the recipe makes enough for a week.

21 grams Huang qi
(astragalus)

9 grams Ling zhi (reishi)

7½ cups water

9 grams Ju hua
(chrysanthemum)

1. Place the Huang qi and Ling zhi in a non-aluminum saucepan and add the water.
2. Bring the mixture to a boil, then simmer uncovered for 25 minutes.
3. Add the Ju hua and simmer for another 5 minutes. Remove from the heat.
4. Strain into a large, 8-cup glass measuring cup. If the total amount is less than 7 cups, add water to bring the decoction to 7 cups total.
5. Set aside ½ cup as the first dose to drink immediately, then refrigerate the rest.
6. Drink ½ cup morning and evening for 1 week. After 7 days, discard any remaining decoction and make a new batch.

Anxiety

Thich Nhat Hanh has a wonderful analogy about how emotions are like flowers, and what you water and attend to grows stronger. I love this analogy, but I also know how challenging it can be in some areas of your life to avoid frustration, anxiety, and anger. Chinese herbs can help you spend less time stuck with challenging emotions you'd like to experience less. Anxiety is a condition of the Heart when Blood or Yin deficiency keeps the Shen unsettled. It can feel like anxiety, tension, stress, or nervousness, with physical symptoms such as tightness in the chest, rapid, shallow breathing patterns, or a sensation of palpitations.

Decoction to Calm Anxiety

MAKES 1 CUP

I've had multiple herbal clients report fluttery feelings of palpitation to their doctors ... but nothing shows up on tests. (If this occurs, I still always recommend checking with your health care provider.) Even though these types of palpitations do not show up on Western diagnostic tests, they feel very real when you experience them. Formulas like this one can help. Long yan rou (longan) builds Blood and calms the Shen, while Gou qi zi (goji berry) supports the Shen by further nourishing Blood. Mei gui hua (rosebud) cools and ensures your Qi is flowing smoothly.

4 to 6 pieces Long yan rou (longan)

1 teaspoon Gou qi zi (goji berry)

1½ cups water

4 to 6 buds Mei gui hua (rosebud)

1. Place the Long yan rou and Gou qi zi in a non-aluminum saucepan and add the water.

2. Bring the mixture to a boil, then simmer uncovered for 20 minutes.

3. Add the Mei gui hua and simmer for another 5 minutes. Remove from the heat.

4. Strain and drink. Repeat up to 3 times per day. You can triple the batch and drink throughout the day.

Decoction to Cool Anxiety

MAKES 1 CUP

He huan hua (albizzia flower) leads this formula to calm the Shen, while Tian men dong (asparagus root) helps cool and ground by building Yin. Da zao (dates) warms and gives digestive strength; Tian men dong can be a heavy, cold herb that can be hard to digest.

1 teaspoon Tian men dong (asparagus root)

1 or 2 pieces Da zao (dates)

1½ cups water

1 tablespoon He huan hua (albizzia flower)

1. Place the Tian men dong and Da zao in a non-aluminum saucepan and add the water.

2. Bring the mixture to a boil, then simmer uncovered for 20 minutes.

3. Add the He huan hua and simmer for another 5 minutes. Remove from the heat.

4. Strain and drink. Repeat up to 3 times a day. You can triple the batch and drink throughout the day.

Decoction to Soothe Anxiety

MAKES 1 CUP

Tongue diagnosis is an important tool in my herbal practice and one we spend a lot of time on when we train students. Anxiety can come with a tip of the tongue that is red and symptoms of heat like flushing in the chest and face or irritability. Dan shen (salvia) cools heat while calming the Shen. Mei gui hua (rosebud) cools and gently moves any blocked Qi, while Da zao (dates) warms and balances the cold temperature of the other two herbs.

2 teaspoons Dan shen
(salvia)

1 or 2 pieces Da zao (dates)

1½ cups water

5 or 6 buds Mei gui hua
(rosebud)

1. Place the Dan shen and Da zao in a non-aluminum saucepan and add the water.

2. Bring the mixture to a boil, then simmer uncovered for 20 minutes.

3. Add the Mei gui hua and simmer for another 5 minutes. Remove from the heat.

4. Strain and drink.

PRECAUTIONS: Do not use Dan shen (salvia) while pregnant or nursing.

Infusion to Promote a Meditative Mind

MAKES 1 CUP

Long yan rou (longan) helps with overthinking. In addition, flowers are good for the heart and Shen. Here, He huan hua (albizzia flower) also calms the Shen, helping you settle into meditation. I have found in addition to nonstop thoughts, Liver Qi stagnation can make it hard to be still, so Mei gui hua (rosebud) is included to smooth the Qi.

5 or 6 buds Mei gui hua (rosebud)

1 tablespoon He huan hua (albizzia flower)

3 or 4 pieces Long yan rou (longan berry)

1½ cups water

1. Place the Mei gui hua, He huan hua, and Long yan rou in a teapot, large mug, or coffee press.

2. Boil the water and pour it over the herbs. Cover and infuse for at least 15 minutes and up to 8 hours.

3. To enjoy during your early morning meditation, infuse the herbs at bedtime so they are ready the next morning, adding more hot water to warm the infusion up.

4. If you like, enjoy the longan berries after they've infused.

Back Pain

The American Chiropractic Association reports that up to 80 percent of Americans will suffer from back pain at some point, causing missed work and medical bills in addition to pain. In Chinese medicine, back pain can be caused by stagnation and Heat or inflammation, or weakness and Cold leading to strains and aches. Discerning the pattern will help indicate which herbs are most appropriate. Sharp, stabbing pain that may dislike pressure indicates stagnation. Heat and pressure will help back pain resulting from deficiency and Cold, and the pain will be more achy and weak feeling.

Decoction for Back and Knee Pain

MAKES 7 CUPS

This formula is for pain that feels weak, loves heat and pressure, and can feel achy instead of sharp and stabbing. Xu duan (teasel) is excellent for lower-back pain, because of its affinity for that part of the body and for warming and building the Yang to strengthen the lower body. Huang qi (astragalus) supports Xu duan by lifting the Yang, and Rou gui (cinnamon bark) assists by warming the Yang. Dan shen (salvia) balances the heat with cool, moving properties.

21 grams Xu duan (teasel)

15 grams Huang qi (astragalus)

9 grams Dan shen (salvia)

7½ cups water

9 grams Rou gui (cinnamon bark)

1. Place the Xu duan, Huang qi, and Dan shen in a non-aluminum saucepan and add the water.
2. Bring the mixture to a boil, then simmer uncovered for 25 minutes. Remove from the heat.
3. Strain into a large, 8-cup glass measuring cup. If the total amount is less than 7 cups, add water to the decoction to bring it to 7 cups total.
4. Add the Rou gui to the strained decoction.
5. Set aside ½ cup as the first dose to drink immediately, then refrigerate the rest.
6. Drink ½ cup morning and evening for 1 week. After 7 days, discard any remaining decoction and make a new batch.

Herbal Oil for Back and Lower-Body Pain

MAKES ONE 16-OUNCE BOTTLE

This is a warming, nourishing formula that addresses Yang deficiency and Cold. This type of pain will not have redness and loves heat, like a heating pad. Xu duan (teasel) is warming and tonifies the Yang, while Huang qi (astragalus) lifts Qi and Spleen Yang. Dan shen (salvia) is cooling and moving, and Gui zhi (cinnamon twig) is warming and moving. Yang deficiency is a cold condition, so the warming herbs help build Yang and alleviate pain caused by Yang deficiency and Cold.

2 tablespoons Xu duan (teasel)

1 tablespoon Dan shen (salvia)

1 tablespoon Gui zhi (cinnamon twig)

1 teaspoon Huang qi (astragalus)

1 teaspoon Xiao hui xiang (fennel)

3 to 5 Yi zhi ren (cardamom) pods

14 ounces oil of your choice

1. Fill a 16-ounce glass container with the Xu duan, Dan shen, Gui zhi, Huang qi, Xiao hui xiang, and Yi zhi ren, leaving space between the top of the herbs and the top of the jar.

2. Cover completely with the oil and secure the lid. It is important that no herbs are above the oil and remain uncovered, as this can ruin the oil.

3. Let the oil sit for 6 weeks, then strain and store in a glass container. The oil will keep in the refrigerator for up to 6 months to a year.

4. Use 1 to 3 tablespoons for massage of the lower back, knees, ankles, or feet. This oil can be gently warmed before applying.

Liniment for Back and Lower-Body Pain

MAKES ONE 16-OUNCE BOTTLE

This is the same basic formula as the Herbal Oil for Back and Lower-Body Pain but designed to be made into a liniment.

2 tablespoons Xu duan (teasel)

1 tablespoon Dan shen (salvia)

1 tablespoon Gui zhi (cinnamon twig)

1 teaspoon Huang qi (astragalus)

1 teaspoon Xiao hui xiang (fennel)

2 pods Yi zhi ren (cardamom)

14 ounces vodka or alcohol of your choice

1. Fill a 16-ounce glass container with the Xu duan, Dan shen, Gui zhi, Huang qi, Xiao hui xiang, and Yi zhi ren, leaving at least 2 inches between the top of the herbs and the top of the jar.

2. Fill the jar to the top with alcohol, making sure it completely covers the herbs, then secure the lid.

3. Infuse the herbs in the alcohol for at least 6 weeks, shaking it daily (or as often as you remember) to mix all the ingredients.

4. After 6 weeks have passed, strain the herbs and store the liniment in a glass container out of the sun. Alcohol extractions like this liniment can be used for up to 3 years if stored somewhere dark and cool.

5. Liniments dry quickly and need frequent application. Use enough liniment to cover the injured area, massaging the affected area if desired. Apply multiple times throughout the day.

Blood Deficiencies

Blood deficiency is common and can happen at any age, although it is more common at times of heavy menstruation and childbirth. Symptoms of Blood deficiency include a pale complexion, floaters in the visual field, muscle cramping, low-grade muscle tension, feeling tired, dizziness, and dry skin.

Syrup for Building Blood

MAKES ONE 16-OUNCE BOTTLE

My first experience making a Blood-building syrup was Todd Caldecott's recipe from his book *Food as Medicine*. I've made many variations on his original recipe, and as a syrup it is a sweet, easy medicinal to add into your day. In this recipe, the Yi zhi ren (cardamom) and Xiao hui xiang (fennel) are included to help digest the sweeter, denser tonic fruits and herbs. The berries and Bai shao (peony) all build Blood. The Huang qi (astragalus) is included to build Qi, which supports the building of Blood. You can take a spoonful twice a day or add it as a topping to dishes like oatmeal. This Blood-building syrup is excellent for any signs or symptoms of Blood deficiency, and can also be used to rebuild after donating blood or postpartum. It is a true tonic, so consistently taking it over a long period of time yields the best results.

½ cup Gou qi zi (goji berry)

½ cup Sang shen (mulberry)

½ cup Long yan rou (longan)

½ cup Da zao (dates)

40 grams Bai shao (peony)

30 grams Huang qi (astragalus)

20 grams Shan zha (hawthorn)

8 cups water

1. Place the Gou qi zi, Sang shen, Long yan rou, Da zao, Bai shao, Huang qi, and Shan zha in a large, non-aluminum stockpot and add the water.

2. Bring the mixture to a boil, then simmer until the liquid is thick, stirring occasionally. After 45 minutes, check the thickness of the liquid (this can be cooked for up to 90 minutes). When the liquid begins to look syrupy, remove from the heat and cool.

3. Before straining the mixture, use a blender, food processor, or potato masher to smash up the fruits and herbs to extract all of the rich juices and liquid from them.

Syrup for Building Blood *continued*

2 tablespoons water, ghee, or coconut oil

1 teaspoon Xiao hui xiang (fennel)

1 to 2 teaspoons Yi zhi ren (cardamom) seeds, crushed

Molasses

4. Place the Gou qi zi, Sang shen, Long yan rou, Da zao, Bai shao, Huang qi, and Shan zha in a large, non-aluminum stockpot and add the water.

5. Bring the mixture to a boil, then simmer until the liquid is thick, stirring occasionally. After 45 minutes, check the thickness of the liquid (this can be cooked for up to 90 minutes). When the liquid begins to look syrupy, remove from the heat and cool.

6. Before straining the mixture, use a blender, food processor, or potato masher to smash up the fruits and herbs to extract all of the rich juices and liquid from them.

7. Using a large, fine-mesh strainer, press out the mixture into an 8-cup glass measuring cup. If the mixture is thick, use a spoon or spatula to help press it through the strainer.

8. Make a note of how much syrupy decoction is in the measuring cup. You will need to measure out the same amount of molasses for a 1:1 ratio to make the syrup (it takes that much sugar to preserve the decoction).

9. Into the now-empty stockpot, place the 2 tablespoons of water, ghee, or coconut oil and add the Xiao hui xiang and crushed Yi zhi ren. Simmer for 1 to 2 minutes, then add the syrupy decoction back to the stockpot and stir to combine. Add equal parts molasses and stir to blend completely. Continue to stir and cook on low heat for 10 minutes, then remove from the heat.

10. Syrups are best stored in a glass container like a mason jar. This can be stored in a cool, dry place or the refrigerator. Tonic formulas like this syrup should be taken daily and used within 6 months. Strain a second time as you pour into your storage bottle.

11. Take 1 to 2 tablespoons per day, with warm water or mixed in with food like a smoothie or oatmeal.

Fruit Blend with Blood-Building Herbs

MAKES 2 TO 3 SERVINGS

Cooked fruits are warming and welcoming, especially in the autumn and winter. This recipe is for a nourishing fruit blend you can enjoy warm on dishes like oatmeal. Feel free to add a favorite fruit or a teaspoon of cinnamon powder.

2 tablespoons Gou qi zi (goji berry)

2 tablespoons Sang shen (mulberry)

2 tablespoons Da zao (dates)

1 tablespoon Shan zha (hawthorn)

1 teaspoon Yi zhi ren (cardamom) seeds, crushed (or 8 to 10 whole pods, crushed)

2½ cups of water

1. Place the Gou qi zi, Sang shen, Da zao, Shan zha, and Yi zhi ren in a non-aluminum saucepan and add the water.

2. Bring the mixture to a boil, then simmer for 10 minutes, stirring frequently. Some of the water should evaporate, and the mixture will thicken, but you don't want it to scorch. Add more water by the tablespoon if needed. Remove from the heat.

3. Leave the fruits whole or blend for a compote-like consistency. Add ½ cup warm blend to dishes like oatmeal or quinoa. Refrigerate leftovers and eat within 3 days.

Blood-Building Herbs for Smoothies

MAKES ½ CUP

This formula increases the nutrition and digestibility of your daily smoothie, plus the Yi zhi ren (cardamom) warms the cold food and helps with digestion. Try omitting the ice in your smoothies and adding warm water instead. Gou qi zi (goji berry) builds Blood, and Huang qi (astragalus) builds the Qi necessary to make Blood.

1 tablespoon Huang qi (astragalus)

½ teaspoon Yi zhi ren (cardamom) seeds, crushed

1 cup water

3 tablespoons Gou qi zi (goji berry)

1. Place the Huang qi and Yi zhi ren in a non-aluminum saucepan and add the water. Simmer covered for 20 minutes, then remove from the heat. Strain and save the decoction.

2. Soak the Gou qi zi in the decoction overnight in a glass container with lid. (Note: If the Gou qi zi soaks up all of the decoction, add more water to just cover. In general, 3 tablespoons of dried fruit can absorb ½ cup of water.)

3. Add the Gou qi zi and soaking liquid to your smoothie.

4. This recipe can be made for 5 days by multiplying the ingredients by five, following the same instructions, and storing in the refrigerator to add to smoothies over 5 days. Use about 4 tablespoons of soaked goji berries per day.

Blood Pressure

While hypertension is often seen as idiopathic in Western medicine, meaning the cause is unknown, Chinese medicine sees hypertension as a symptom with multiple underlying patterns of disharmony that can be clearly identified. From Wind to Yin deficiency to Heat and stagnation, determining the full view of the patterns of disharmony can help.

Decoction for High Blood Pressure

MAKES 7 CUPS

Many calming herbs can help lower blood pressure, including the herbal formulas for anxiety and frustration. This formula helps with hypertension by anchoring Wind, clearing Heat, and building Yin. It is very similar to the migraine formulas, because high blood pressure can cause headaches and has the same pattern basis as migraines in Chinese medicine: Internal Liver Wind.

12 grams Bai shao (peony)

9 grams Xu duan (teasel)

9 grams Da zao (dates)

6 grams Tian men dong (asparagus root)

6 grams Mu dan pi (tree peony)

8 cups water

21 grams Gou teng (cat's claw)

6 grams Ju hua (chrysanthemum)

1. Place the Bai shao, Xu duan, Da zao, Tian men dong, and Mu dan pi in a non-aluminum saucepan and add the water.

2. Bring the mixture to a boil, then simmer uncovered for 25 minutes.

3. Add the Gou teng and Ju hua and simmer for another 5 minutes. Remove from the heat.

4. Strain into a large, 8-cup glass measuring cup. If the total amount is less than 7 cups, add water to the decoction to bring it to 7 cups total.

5. Set aside ½ cup as the first dose to drink immediately, then refrigerate the rest.

6. Drink ½ cup morning and evening for 1 week. After 7 days, discard any remaining decoction.

PRECAUTIONS: Communicate with your doctor and monitor your blood pressure. Herbal medicines can mutually enhance the actions of medications to lower blood pressure.

Blood Sugar

Elevated blood-sugar levels should first inspire evaluation of diet and lifestyle, including sleep habits and stress levels. Herbal medicine can help further manage blood sugar. Many herbs can lower blood sugar as they help bring the body into balance, building digestive strength and fostering deeper sleep and better stress management.

Diabetes-Friendly Infusion of Fenugreek

MAKES 1 CUP

There are two methods to prepare fenugreek seeds, which are very hard and must be cooked before eating. The first is to soak the Hu lu ba (fenugreek) overnight in water; the second decocts the Hu lu ba, which softens the fenugreek more. Fenugreek is a good source of fiber, so there is a benefit to consuming the whole seed.

1 tablespoon Hu lu ba
  (fenugreek)

1½ cups water

SOAKING METHOD:

1. Place the Hu lu ba in a bowl or glass jar and add the water.
2. Cover and soak overnight.
3. Strain and drink before one or all meals.

DECOCTION METHOD:

1. Place the Hu lu ba in a non-aluminum saucepan and add the water.
2. Bring the mixture to a boil, and then simmer uncovered for 10 minutes. Remove from the heat.
3. Do not strain the mixture; soak the Hu lu ba decoction for a few hours or overnight.
4. Drink the decoction, including the soaked seeds if desired. The soaked seeds can also be eaten or added to dishes.

Diabetes-Friendly Cinnamon Tea

MAKES 1 CUP

Research supports cinnamon's many health benefits, including managing blood sugar and type 2 diabetes. You can use ground cinnamon or the cinnamon you find at your herbal apothecary: Gui zhi (cinnamon twig) and Rou gui (cinnamon bark). I personally find the flavor of Rou gui stronger than that of Gui zhi. It is more warming and building, while Gui zhi is more moving. I use Rou gui over Gui zhi to make this cinnamon beverage for regular use, but you can try either. This makes for a wonderful beverage during colder weather. It could also be mixed with an apple fruit tea for a sugarless apple cider-style drink.

1 to 2 teaspoons Rou gui (cinnamon bark)

1¼ cups water or other beverage of choice (e.g., oat milk or apple fruit tea)

1⅛ teaspoons vanilla extract (optional)

1. Place the Rou gui (or Gui zhi or powdered cinnamon) in a non-aluminum saucepan and add your beverage of choice.

2. Simmer gently, stirring, until well mixed and heated through, about 5 minutes. Remove from the heat and steep for another 5 minutes so the cinnamon can further infuse into the hot liquid.

3. Strain and add the vanilla if desired. Drink warm.

Breast Health

In qigong, the Chinese energy practice, the area around the breast is included in practices to keep Qi and lymph circulating. Here, Chinese herbs help maintain breast health through promoting healthy Qi and fluid circulation.

Herbal Oil for Breast Health

MAKES ONE 16-OUNCE BOTTLE

The herbs in this oil circulate Qi and fluids in the chest. Good for overall breast health, it can also help with breast tenderness as a part of PMS. Gui zhi (cinnamon twig) is warming, and Mei gui hua (rosebud) is cooling. Both help circulate Qi, while massaging in the oil circulates lymph. Having a routine helps remind you to perform regular breast checks. Using the recipes in chapter 2 (page 19), you can also make this oil into a salve if that consistency is preferable.

28 grams Mei gui hua (rosebud)

14 grams Tian men dong (asparagus root)

14 grams Gui zhi (cinnamon twig)

14 ounces oil of your choice

1. Fill a 16-ounce glass container with the Mei gui hua, Tian men dong, and Gui zhi, leaving space between the top of the herbs and the top of the jar.

2. Cover completely with the oil and secure the lid. It is important that no herbs are above the oil and remain uncovered, as this can ruin the oil.

3. Let the oil sit for 6 weeks, then strain and store in a glass container. The oil will keep in the refrigerator for up to 6 months to a year.

4. Massage a small amount on breasts daily—for example, immediately after a shower or before bed, when you can allow 5 to 10 minutes for the oil to fully absorb before getting dressed.

Breast-Milk Production

Breast-milk supply can sometimes use a boost, and there are herbs called galactagogues that can help increase milk levels.

Decoction to Increase Milk Supply

MAKES 1 CUP

Hu lu ba (fenugreek) and Xiao hui xiang (fennel) are both galactagogues, meaning they support breast-milk production. They can be used alone, but Mei gui hua (rosebud) makes for a helpful addition by calming and moving Qi. There are energy meridians that go through the breast area, and opening them can help with production. This works well in conjunction with Postpartum Syrup (page 162) to build Qi and Blood. Consistent dosing is needed for best results.

2 teaspoons Hu lu ba (fenugreek)

2 teaspoons Xiao hui xiang (fennel)

1½ cups water

2 or 3 buds Mei gui hua (rosebud)

1. Place the Hu lu ba and Xiao hui xiang in a non-aluminum saucepan and add the water.

2. Bring the mixture to a boil, then simmer uncovered for 20 minutes. Remove from heat and add the Mei gui hua. Allow to infuse for 30 minutes.

3. Strain and drink. You can triple the ingredients to make one larger batch, keeping it in a thermos to drink warm throughout the day. Refrigerate any leftovers for use the next day, remembering to warm the decoction before drinking. Discard leftovers after 48 hours. Repeat up to 3 times per day.

Cholesterol

Excess Dampness and stagnation can be underlying patterns for cholesterol issues. To lower and optimize cholesterol, your digestion needs to be strong. Along with herbs specifically for cholesterol, correcting other patterns of disharmony like Heat, Cold, stagnation, or deficiencies like Qi or Blood deficiency further supports healthy cholesterol levels.

Decoction for Cholesterol Management

MAKES 7 CUPS

These three herbs help with digestion and have research supporting their use to help manage cholesterol. Because cholesterol management requires long-term support, it is best to stay consistent and consume this decoction daily for at least three months and ideally until your cholesterol is checked again.

½ cup Shan zha (hawthorn)

5 tablespoons Hu lu ba (fenugreek)

5 tablespoons Xiao hui xiang (fennel)

8 cups water

1. Place the Shan zha, Hu lu ba, and Xiao hui xiang in a non-aluminum saucepan and add the water.

2. Bring the mixture to a boil, then simmer uncovered for 20 minutes. Add ¼ cup water if needed due to the herbs absorbing a lot. Remove from the heat.

3. Strain into a large, 8-cup glass measuring cup. If the total amount is less 7 cups, add water to the decoction to bring it to 7 cups total.

4. Set aside ½ cup as the first dose to drink immediately, then refrigerate the rest.

5. Drink ½ cup morning and evening for 1 week. After 7 days, discard any remaining decoction and make a new batch.

Colds and Flu

In Chinese medicine, colds are the result of External Wind getting through our usual defenses and becoming "Internal." Symptoms vary depending on the individual, their constitution, existing imbalances, and even their environment. A person living in the warm, humid South may have more Dampness with a cold, while someone living in the mountains or desert may have more symptoms of dryness. We can modify cold formulas to be more helpful depending on how each person is sick. It is best to begin taking these cold formulas at the first sign of a cold, before you are really in the thick of it. This is where being mindful of your body helps, because you will learn to identify your "first sign." For some, it is in the throat (a scratch, a tickle); for others, it's more about the nose and congestion.

A tip for cold remedies: When you are sick, it can be a challenge to prepare remedies multiple times per day. One solution is to make a double or triple batch and put it in a thermos so you can drink the warm decoction slowly throughout the day. If the mixture gets cold, do not microwave it; instead, add hot water to warm it.

Decoction for Colds

MAKES 1 CUP

This formula will help ease the symptoms of a cold or, in Chinese energetic terms, "release it to the exterior." The Gui zhi (cinnamon twig) is warming and circulating and releases exterior Cold. The Bai shao (peony) works with the Gui zhi to help with chills and fever, mild sweating, and other symptoms of a head cold. Da zao (dates) helps boost Qi to help fight off the illness.

2 teaspoons Gui zhi (cinnamon twig)

1 teaspoon Bai shao (peony)

1 large or 2 small Da zao (dates)

1½ cups water

1. Place the Gui zhi, Bai shao, and Da zao in a non-aluminum saucepan and add the water. Bring the mixture to a boil, then simmer uncovered for 20 minutes. Remove from the heat.

2. Strain and drink the decoction over the next half hour. Repeat up to 3 times a day.

PRECAUTIONS: This decoction is not for long-term use.

Decoction for a Cold with a Fever

MAKES 1 CUP

This remedy is for an External invasion or a cold/flu with more Heat, presenting as a fever, a sensation of feeling hot, red eyes, and a sore, painful throat.

2 teaspoons Bo he (mint)

2 teaspoons Ju hua (chrysanthemum)

1½ cups water

1. Place the Bo he and Ju hua in a non-aluminum saucepan and add the water.

2. Bring the mixture to a boil, then simmer uncovered for 20 minutes. Remove from the heat.

3. Strain and drink the decoction over the next half hour. Repeat up to 3 times a day.

PRECAUTIONS: This decoction is not for long-term use.

Decoction for a Cold with Neck and Shoulder Stiffness

MAKES 1 CUP

This remedy is for an External invasion when a major accompanying symptom is muscle tightness and stiffness, usually in your neck and shoulders. It uses the combination of Gui zhi (cinnamon twig) to release the exterior condition and help fight the cold and Ge gen (kudzu) to help release exterior conditions while relaxing and releasing tension in the upper body. Bai shao (peony) supports both of those herbs in their actions.

2 teaspoons Gui zhi
(cinnamon twig)

2 teaspoons Ge gen (kudzu)

1 teaspoon Bai
shao (peony)

1½ cups water

1. Place the Gui zhi, Ge gen, and Bai shao in a non-aluminum saucepan and add the water.

2. Bring the mixture to a boil, then simmer uncovered for 20 minutes. Remove from the heat.

3. Strain and drink the decoction over the next half hour. Repeat up to 3 times a day.

PRECAUTIONS: This decoction is not for long-term use.

Decoction for a Cold with Headache

MAKES 1 CUP

Chuan xiong (ligusticum) is a helpful herb for headaches. This formula is for headaches that come with a cold or flu. It can be used alone, or it can be alternated with another formula for different symptoms.

2 teaspoons Gui zhi (cinnamon twig)

2 teaspoons Chuan xiong (ligusticum)

1½ cups water

1. Place the Gui zhi and Chuan xiong in a non-aluminum saucepan and add the water.

2. Bring the mixture to a boil, then simmer uncovered for 20 minutes. Remove from the heat.

3. Strain and drink the decoction over the next half hour. Repeat up to 3 times a day.

PRECAUTIONS: Do not use Chuan xiong while pregnant or nursing unless under the care of a licensed practitioner.

Decoction for a Cold with Body Aches

MAKES 1 CUP

Adding on to the basic cold formula, Du huo (angelica) and Ge gen (kudzu) help with aches and pain and tension that can come with an External invasion.

2 teaspoons Du huo (angelica)

1 teaspoon Gui zhi (cinnamon twig)

1 teaspoon Bai shao (peony)

1 teaspoon Ge gen (kudzu)

1½ cups water

1. Place the Du huo, Gui zhi, Bai shao, and Ge gen in a non-aluminum saucepan and add the water.

2. Bring the mixture to a boil, then simmer uncovered for 20 minutes. Remove from the heat.

3. Strain and drink the decoction over the next half hour. Repeat up to 3 times a day.

PRECAUTIONS: This decoction is not for long-term use.

Decoction for a Cold with Cough

MAKES 1 CUP

Zi wan (aster) is added here to help with the cough that comes with a cold. Not too hot or too cold, it can also be used for a general cough.

2 teaspoons Gui zhi (cinnamon twig)

1 teaspoon Bai shao (peony)

1 small Da zao (dates)

1½ cups water

2 teaspoons Zi wan (aster)

1. Place the Gui zhi, Bai shao, and Da zao in a non-aluminum saucepan and add the water.

2. Bring the mixture to a boil, then simmer for 20 minutes.

3. Add the Zi wan, and simmer uncovered for another 5 minutes. Remove from the heat.

4. Strain and drink the decoction over the next half hour. Repeat up to 3 times a day.

PRECAUTIONS: This decoction is not for long-term use.

Decoction for a Cold with a Fever and Cough

MAKES 1 CUP

Gua lou (tricosanthes) strengthens this formula to be even more geared toward coughs, especially a cough that is productive, with phlegm and nasal congestion. Gua lou has a stronger effect on draining and transforming the phlegm.

2 teaspoons Zi wan (aster)

1 teaspoon Gua lou (tricosanthes)

1½ cups water

1 teaspoon Ju hua (chrysanthemum)

1. Place the Zi wan and Gua loa in a non-aluminum saucepan and add the water.

2. Bring the mixture to a boil, then simmer uncovered for 20 minutes.

3. Add the Ju hua, and simmer uncovered for another 10 minutes. Remove from the heat.

4. Strain and drink the decoction over the next half hour. Repeat up to 3 times a day.

PRECAUTIONS: This decoction is not for long-term use. Do not use Gua lou during pregnancy or nursing unless under the care of a licensed practitioner.

Decoction for a Cold with a Dry Cough

MAKES 1 CUP

With or without a cold, a dry, hacking cough is tiring and uncomfortable. This formula moistens the Lungs to help with the pain and tightness that come with the dryness, while the Ju hua (chrysanthemum) and Zi wan (aster) help release to the exterior and alleviate the cough. A little honey can be added to soothe a throat raw from coughing.

2 teaspoons Mai men dong (ophiopogon)

1 teaspoon Zi wan (aster)

1½ cups water

1 teaspoon Bo he (mint)

1 teaspoon Ju hua (chrysanthemum)

1. Place the Mai men dong and Zi wan in a non-aluminum saucepan and add the water.

2. Bring the mixture to a boil, then simmer uncovered for 20 minutes.

3. Add the Bo he and Ju hua, and simmer uncovered for another 10 minutes. Remove from the heat.

4. Strain and drink the decoction over the next half hour. Repeat up to 3 times a day.

PRECAUTIONS: This decoction is not for long-term use. If a cough persists for more than a few weeks, reevaluate the patterns to update the formula. Consult your doctor for persistent coughs that do not improve.

Decoction for a Cold with Mucus

MAKES 1 CUP

Fu ling (poria) addresses a cold with clear or white watery mucus by draining the Dampness. Gui zhi (cinnamon twig) also helps with Dampness due to its warmth and movement.

2 teaspoons Gui zhi (cinnamon twig)

2 teaspoons Fu ling (poria)

1½ cups water

1. Place the Gui zhi and Fu ling in a non-aluminum saucepan and add the water.

2. Bring the mixture to a boil, then simmer uncovered for 30 minutes. Remove from the heat.

3. Strain and drink the decoction over the next half hour. Repeat up to 3 times a day.

Constipation

As with everything in Chinese herbal medicine, one condition can have various causes. Constipation is no different. To distinguish between the causes of constipation, you need to look at the condition of your stool after it passes, your patterns and temperature overall, and if anything makes it better or worse. Normal bowel movements should be daily and not painful.

Constipation can be from Qi and Yang deficiency when there isn't enough energy sometimes to pass stool, but when it does, it is not always dry and can be a normal-looking bowel movement. More frequently, constipation is due to a deficiency of fluids, Blood, or Yin.

Decoction to Moisten Constipation

MAKES 7 CUPS

This is a general formula for constipation with stools that can be dry and hard to pass. In Chinese herbal medicine, along with Yin and Blood tonics, seeds like flaxseed are also moistening and beneficial for treating constipation. Herbs like senna help empty the bowels but do not treat the underlying conditions causing the constipation and can also become habit-forming. This formula treats the root of the problem and should be taken daily to build up fluids and Yin to balance elimination.

30 grams Mai men dong (ophiopogon)

24 grams Gou qi zi (goji berry)

12 grams Da zao (dates)

3 grams Yi zhi ren (cardamom)

8 cups water

1. Place the Mai men dong, Gou qi zi, Da zao, and Yi zhi ren in a non-aluminum stockpot and add the water.

2. Bring the mixture to a boil, then simmer uncovered for 30 minutes. Remove from the heat.

3. Strain into a large, 8-cup glass measuring cup. If the total amount is less than 7 cups, add water to bring the decoction to 7 cups total.

4. Set aside ½ cup as the first dose to drink immediately, then refrigerate the rest.

5. Drink ½ cup morning and evening for 1 week. After 7 days, discard any remaining decoction and make a new batch.

Decoction for Constipation with Heat

MAKES 7 CUPS

If there are significant signs of Heat along with the dryness, 12 grams of Gua lou ren (tricosanthes seed) can be added to the previous formula to further clear Heat. Symptoms include feeling warm, especially at night, night sweats, and very dry stools. Dryness could also be more severe, with thirst, dry skin and hair, and possible red rashes on the skin. Gua lou ren is further moistening and cooling, strengthening those effects of the base formula for constipation.

30 grams Mai men dong (ophiopogon)

24 grams Gou qi zi (goji berry)

12 grams Da zao (dates)

12 grams Gua lou ren (tricosanthes seed)

3 grams Yi zhi ren (cardamom)

8 cups water

1. Place the Mai men dong, Gou qi zi, Da zao, Gua lou ren, and Yi zhi ren in a non-aluminum stockpot and add the water.

2. Bring the mixture to a boil, then simmer uncovered for 30 minutes. Remove from the heat.

3. Strain into a large, 8-cup glass measuring cup. If the total amount is less than 7 cups, add water to bring the decoction to 7 cups total.

4. Set aside ½ cup as the first dose to drink immediately, then refrigerate the rest.

5. Drink ½ cup morning and evening for 1 week. After 7 days, discard any remaining decoction and make a new batch.

PRECAUTIONS: Do not use Gua lou ren during pregnancy or nursing unless under the care of a licensed practitioner.

Cough

Coughs can have different patterns of disharmony but commonly are part of a cold, flu, or exterior condition. Depending on factors like individual constitution and environment, a cough can take on different forms. From dry to wet, from feverish and hot with colored mucus to cold with clear mucus, different types of cough are helped by different herbs.

Infusion for Quick Wet-Cough Relief

MAKES 1 CUP

I believe formulas are best, with the herbs acting as members of a team that support and help one another. But sometimes you're sick and tired, and you just need something to help. For a productive cough, for those times you're coughing yourself awake all night, Gua lou (tricosanthes) can be made into a quick tea to help settle the cough. Then, when you've slept and it's daylight again, you can worry about making a more involved formula. Gua lou works well for coughs with mucus but also when breathing is hard and your chest feels heavy. For a wet cough, honey may not be the best, but it can soothe a throat that is rough and scratched from coughing.

1 tablespoon Gua lou (tricosanthes)—smaller pieces are better

1¼ cups water

Honey and lemon (optional)

1. Place the Gua lou in a large mug (or teapot or coffee press).
2. Boil the water and pour it over the herbs. Steep for 20 to 30 minutes.
3. Strain and drink. Repeat up to 3 times a day, adding honey and lemon if desired.

PRECAUTIONS: Do not use Gua lou during pregnancy or nursing unless under the care of a licensed practitioner.

Infusion for Quick Warming Cough Relief

MAKES 1 CUP

For a drier cough, Zi wan (aster) can be used for a quick cup of relief for coughing, especially when the cough is dry. When you are too exhausted to find and make a whole formula, Zi wan can help. Honey can further soothe your throat when it's scratchy and sore from coughing.

1 tablespoon Zi wan (aster)

1¼ cups water

Honey and lemon (optional)

1. Place the Zi wan in a large mug (or teapot or coffee press).

2. Boil the water and pour it over the herbs. Steep for 20 to 30 minutes.

3. Strain and drink. Repeat up to 3 times a day, adding honey and lemon if desired.

Decoction for a Dry Cough

MAKES 7 CUPS

Mai men dong (ophiopogon) moistens and tonifies the Yin of the Lung. Ling zhi (reishi) helps with the Lung Qi, while Bai zhu (atractylodes) tonifies Spleen and Lung Qi and helps dry excess Dampness. Fu ling (poria) assists with the drying of excess fluids. Da zao (dates) is moistening and is one of the "three sweets" to help digest and assimilate the formula. This formula is not the same as Mai Men Dong Tang (Ophiopogon Decoction) but is based on it, using Mai men dong to moisten Lung Yin, with additional herbs to support the Qi of the Lungs and Spleen and fluid metabolism.

18 grams Mai men dong (ophiopogon)

12 pieces Da zao (dates)

12 grams Bai zhu (atractylodes)

6 grams Fu ling (poria)

6 grams Ling zhi (reishi)

8 cups water

1. Place the Mai men dong, Da zao, Bai zhu, Fu ling, and Ling zhi in a non-aluminum saucepan and add the water.

2. Bring the mixture to a boil, then simmer uncovered for 25 minutes. Remove from the heat.

3. Strain into a large, 8-cup glass measuring cup. If the total amount is less than 7 cups, add water to the decoction to bring it to 7 cups total.

4. Set aside ½ cup as the first dose to drink immediately, then refrigerate the rest.

5. Drink ½ cup morning and evening for 1 week. After 7 days, discard any remaining decoction and make a new batch.

Syrup for a Dry Cough

MAKES ONE 16-OUNCE BOTTLE

Zi wan (aster) and Gua lou (tricosanthes) stop coughing, while Gui zhi (cinnamon twig) brings warmth, increases circulation, and helps with any other head-cold symptoms. Mai men dong (ophiopogon) moistens the Lungs and cough, easing dryness.

4 cups water

½ cup Gua lou (tricosanthes)

½ cup Mai men dong (ophiopogon)

½ cup Chen pi (tangerine peel)

½ cup Zi wan (aster)

2 teaspoons Gui zhi (cinnamon twig)

Molasses

1. Place the water in a non-aluminum saucepan and add the Gua lou and Mai men dong.

2. Bring the mixture to a boil, then simmer uncovered for 30 minutes. Add the Chen pi, Zi wan, and Gui zhi. Continue to simmer until the liquid is thick, stirring occasionally. After 45 minutes, check the thickness of the liquid (this can be cooked for up to 60 minutes). When the liquid begins to look syrupy, remove from the heat and cool.

3. Using a fine-mesh strainer, strain the mixture into a large, 8-cup glass measuring cup.

4. Make a note of how much syrupy decoction is in the measuring cup. You will need to measure out the same amount of molasses for a 1:1 ratio to make the syrup.

5. Return the syrup to the saucepan, add equal parts molasses, and stir to blend completely. Continue to stir and simmer for 10 minutes, then remove from heat.

6. Store in a glass container in a cool, dry place or the refrigerator for up to 6 months.

7. Take 1 to 2 teaspoons as needed.

PRECAUTIONS: Do not use Gua lou during pregnancy or nursing unless under the care of a licensed practitioner.

Syrup for a Wet Cough

MAKES ONE 16-OUNCE BOTTLE

For a wet cough, Gua Lou (tricosanthes) deals with a productive cough, while Fu ling (poria) assists in fluid management, draining it. Chen pi (tangerine peel) and Gui zhi (cinnamon twig) warm and move, and Gui zhi also helps with any head-cold symptoms.

4 cups water

½ cup Fu ling (poria)

½ cup Gua lou (tricosanthes)

½ cup Chen pi (tangerine peel)

1 tablespoon Gui zhi (cinnamon twig)

Molasses

1. Place the water in a non-aluminum saucepan and add the Fu ling and Gua lou.

2. Bring the mixture to a boil, then simmer uncovered for 30 minutes. Add the Chen pi and Gui zhi. Continue to simmer until the liquid is thick, stirring occasionally. After 45 minutes, check the thickness of the liquid (this can be cooked for up to 60 minutes). When the liquid begins to look syrupy, remove from the heat and cool.

3. Using a fine-mesh strainer, strain the mixture into a large, 8-cup glass measuring cup.

4. Make a note of how much syrupy decoction is in the measuring cup. You will need to measure out the same amount of molasses for a 1:1 ratio to make the syrup.

5. Return the syrup to the saucepan, add equal parts molasses, and stir to blend completely. Continue to stir and simmer for 10 minutes, then remove from the heat.

6. Store in a glass container in a cool, dry place or the refrigerator for up to 6 months.

7. Take 1 to 2 teaspoons as needed.

PRECAUTIONS: Do not use Gua lou during pregnancy.

Dental Health

Long before you could buy toothpaste, floss, and other modern-day dental aids, traditional systems of medicine had ways to clean the mouth and teeth and help maintain dental health.

Mouth Rinse for Tooth Pain

MAKES 2 CUPS

Du huo (angelica) can help with different types of pain. It is found in many formulas both internal and topical for muscle and joint pain. In this remedy, Du huo acts on pain in the teeth and mouth. This isn't fixing the problem but helps alleviate the pain until you can get to the dentist. Did you know there are also acupuncture points specific to tooth pain?

2 tablespoons Du huo (angelica)

2 cups water

1. Place the Du huo in a non-aluminum saucepan and add the water.

2. Bring the mixture to a boil, then simmer uncovered for 20 minutes. Remove from the heat.

3. Strain and use as a mouth rinse. Holding it in your mouth for as long as possible is helpful with pain. Use a few tablespoons to rinse, repeating when necessary.

PRECAUTIONS: This is only for short-term use. Always see a dentist to address the source of your pain.

Mouth Rinse for Dental Health

MAKES 1 CUP

Herbal blends can be used as part of a daily dental health routine, supporting gum health and killing bacteria as well as freshening the breath. I have also used well-strained dental rinses in my water flossing system, like a Waterpik.

2 teaspoons Xiao hui xiang (fennel)

1 teaspoon Jiang huang (turmeric)

3 pods Yi zhi ren (cardamom), crushed

1½ cups water

1. Place the Xiao hui xiang, Jiang huang, and Yi zhi ren in a non-aluminum saucepan and add the water.

2. Bring the mixture to a boil, then simmer uncovered for 20 minutes. Remove from the heat.

3. Strain and use as a mouth rinse. This decoction can be saved in a container with a lid; keep it in the refrigerator. Rinse with 1 to 2 tablespoons after brushing.

4. You can chew on the Yi zhi ren and Xiao hui xiang seeds after they've been decocted if you like the flavor.

Digestion

Digestion is the foundation of health, and formulas that promote healthy digestive function are an aid to all other systems in your body. What you take in, what nourishes you, is used by the Earth element—the Spleen and Stomach—to make Qi that supports your daily activities. Good digestion and caring for yourself is a daily act of healthy living.

Cooking Blend for Digestion

MAKES ¼ CUP

Add this to almost any dish that will be cooked for at least 15 minutes. This can be used for both savory and sweet foods. I like to add it to oatmeal.

3 to 6 pods Yi zhi ren (cardamom), crushed

2 or 3 pieces Da zao (dates)

2 or 3 pieces Shan zha (hawthorn)

1. In a small bowl, mix together the Yi zhi ren, Da zao, and Shan zha.
2. Add to dishes before cooking.

Cooking Blend with Fennel for Digestion

This digestive blend contains Xiao hui xiang (fennel). With so many benefits, it is worth getting used to the flavor of this herb. Try adding it in smaller amounts and working up to the full teaspoon and beyond. For lightly flavored dishes, use less Yi zhi ren (cardamom) than for more heavily flavored dishes.

8 pods Yi zhi ren (cardamom), crushed

1 teaspoon Xiao hui xiang (fennel)

2 or 3 pieces Shan zha (hawthorn)

1. In a small bowl, mix together the Yi zhi ren, Xiao hui xiang, and Shan zha.

2. Add to dishes before cooking.

Decoction for Digestive Strength

MAKES 1 CUP

Xiao hui xiang (fennel) warms the digestive Fire, Shan zha (hawthorn) acts like a digestive enzyme to facilitate digestion, and Bai zhu (atractylodes) strengthens the Spleen Qi to transform and transport fluids. This is a good formula to drink before lunch and dinner to help with digestion, as the energy of the Spleen and Stomach is highest in the morning and lowest in the evening. According to this cycle of energy, it is better to eat larger meals earlier in the day. Try taking this formula daily over a few weeks to strengthen digestion, then reevaluate to see whether you still need it.

1 tablespoon Bai zhu (atractylodes)

2 berries Shan zha (hawthorn)

1 teaspoon Xiao hui xiang (fennel)

1½ cups water

1. Place the Bai zhu, Shan zha, and Xiao hui xiang in a non-aluminum saucepan and add the water.

2. Bring the mixture to a boil, then simmer uncovered for 20 minutes. Remove from the heat.

3. Strain and drink. Repeat up to 3 times per day.

Decoction for Warming Digestion

MAKES 1 CUP

I have heard many American tourists in Europe complain about the lack of cold, iced drinks, but the Europeans have the right idea. Digestion works best if the Stomach and Spleen have a warm environment. Eating cold foods, foods straight out of the refrigerator, smoothies, and drinks with ice can cause excessive Cold in the Stomach and Spleen, showing up as digestive problems like gas, bloating or loose stools, and increased mucus or Dampness. There can also be a sensation of cold and fullness in the abdomen. TCM practitioners refer to it as "refrigerator syndrome." In addition to limiting cold drinks and foods, you can drink this to help combat the Cold. Adjusting the temperature of your diet may eliminate the need for this formula.

2 teaspoons Bai zhu (atractylodes)

1 teaspoon Yi zhi ren (cardamom) seeds or 8 whole pods crushed open

1½ cups water

1. Place the Bai zhu and Yi zhi ren in a non-aluminum saucepan and add the water.

2. Bring the mixture to a boil, then simmer uncovered for 20 minutes. Remove from the heat.

3. Strain and drink up to 3 times per day while simultaneously decreasing the amount of cold food in your diet.

4. Triple the ingredients for a larger batch. Drink throughout the day while decreasing the amount of cold food in your diet.

Decoction of Digestive Bitters

MAKES 1 CUP

Digestive bitters have had a resurgence in popularity in the last decade. Bitter is a flavor lacking in the modern American palate, yet it's vital for health and balance. Bitters stimulate sluggish digestion and can help with many symptoms of slow digestion, including gas, bloating, constipation, and heartburn caused by low acid. Chinese herbal medicine uses Chen pi (tangerine peel), a gentle bitter with a familiar citrus flavor. As a beginning step, you can add this Chen pi decoction to another fruit tea blend, like Citrus Sunrise by Celestial Seasonings. Drink before meals.

2 teaspoons Chen pi (tangerine peel)

1 cup water

1. Place the Chen pi in a non-aluminum saucepan and add the water.
2. Bring the mixture to a boil, then cover and simmer for 10 minutes. Remove from the heat.
3. Strain and drink before meals.

After-Dinner Fennel

MAKES ABOUT 5 SERVINGS

The best example of after-dinner Xiao hui xiang (fennel) is the brightly colored bowl of candied fennel at Indian restaurants. This version is simpler and omits the colored candy pieces while retaining hints of sweetness. Regular granulated sugar is too small to work well in this formula; you need the larger pieces that come labeled as rock sugar. These amounts are approximate, and you'll want just enough sugar to give a tiny bit of sweet flavor to go along with the fennel. Dr. Bharat Aggarwal's book *Healing Spices* lists all of Xiao hui xiang's digestive benefits and includes its benefits for high blood pressure, heart disease, Alzheimer's, and dementia. Modern research is supporting traditional use of Xiao hui xiang (fennel) as part of a daily routine.

3 tablespoons Xiao hui xiang (fennel)

2 teaspoons rock sugar

1. In a small bowl, mix together the Xiao hui xiang and rock sugar.

2. Store in an airtight container. Enjoy a teaspoon or two after meals. If you enjoy this formula or are having an event like a dinner party, you can make a much larger batch using ¾ cup fennel and ⅛ cup rock sugar.

Infused After-Dinner Fennel

MAKES ABOUT 5 SERVINGS

Getting my son to eat plain fennel is a hard sell, and I think After-Dinner Fennel (page 120) can be a challenging taste for Americans. This recipe soaks the fennel so that every piece is a little sweeter and softer. Once you get used to the flavor of Xiao hui xiang (fennel), you can try reducing the amount of sugar in the water or transition to the After-Dinner Fennel recipe.

2 tablespoons hot water

2 teaspoons rock sugar

3 tablespoons Xiao hui xiang (fennel)

1. In a small bowl, combine the hot water and rock sugar. Stir to dissolve the sugar.

2. Add the fennel and soak for an hour. If there is excess water, drain. Store the fennel in an airtight container.

3. Enjoy a pinch after meals and refrigerate any leftovers.

Elimination

Healthy elimination goes along with healthy digestion—we should be moving out what we do not need! You should have daily bowel movements, and they should not be painful. Loose stools, undigested food in stools, and diarrhea that comes with a menstrual cycle is due to weak Spleen Qi and digestive strength.

Decoction for Healthy Elimination

MAKES 1 CUP

This formula has Bai zhu (atractylodes) to build up Spleen Qi, Fu ling (poria) to further help the Spleen by draining excess Dampness, Chen pi (tangerine peel) to ensure the Qi is flowing smoothly, and Yi zhi ren (cardamom) to add a little flavor and warmth for digestion. Cardamom has a calming, balancing effect on the digestive tract and is helpful for both diarrhea and constipation.

2 teaspoons Bai zhu (atractylodes)

1 teaspoon Chen pi (tangerine peel)

1 teaspoon Fu ling (poria)

1 teaspoon Yi zhi ren (cardamom) seeds or 8 whole pods crushed open

1½ cups water

1. Place the Bai zhu, Chen pi, Fu ling, and Yi zhi ren in a non-aluminum saucepan and add the water.

2. Bring the mixture to a boil, then simmer uncovered for 20 minutes. Remove from the heat.

3. Strain and drink. Repeat up to 2 times daily.

Energy

Using coffee or energy drinks is like buying energy with a credit card. You aren't really paying now, but you'll have to eventually. It's much better to do a "cash transaction"—using quality herbs, getting enough sleep, and eating healthy food. Even the best herbal formula shouldn't be used in place of good lifestyle choices. A perfect example is my patient who came in feeling tired, lethargic, and low on energy. He was healthy overall, but he admitted to watching Netflix in bed, often forgoing sleep to watch one more episode. In the end, I did not give him a formula initially, asking him instead to try a two-week experiment. He would try going to bed earlier, limiting the Netflix, and making sure he was in bed 8 to 10 hours each night whether he was sleeping the whole time or not. He never came to get the formula—after two weeks of good sleep, he didn't need it.

Spleen Qi Decoction (Based on Liu jun zi tang, Six Gentleman Decoction)

MAKES 7 CUPS

This formula can help with energy, but plenty of sleep and nutritious food are also essential to having enough energy.

21 grams Bai zhu (atractylodes)

18 grams Ling zhi (reishi)

15 grams Chen pi (tangerine peel)

12 grams Fu ling (poria)

12 grams Da zao (dates)

7½ cups water

1. Place the Bai zhu, Ling zhi, Chen pi, Fu ling, and Da zao in a non-aluminum stockpot and add the water.

2. Bring the mixture to a boil, then simmer uncovered for 30 minutes. Remove from the heat.

3. Strain into a large, 8-cup glass measuring cup. If the total amount is less than 7 cups, add water to bring it to 7 cups total.

4. Set aside ½ cup as the first dose to drink immediately, then refrigerate the rest.

5. Drink ½ cup morning and evening for 1 week. After 7 days, discard any remaining decoction and make a new batch.

Decoction for Afternoon Energy

MAKES 1 CUP

Having a variety of formulas on hand can be helpful for increasing energy. When you need an afternoon pick-me-up and are craving sugar or caffeine, try this duo of herbs. Bai zhu (atractylodes) is the hardworking Spleen Qi builder, while Chen pi gets the Qi moving.

1 tablespoon Bai zhu (atractylodes)

2 teaspoons Chen pi (tangerine peel)

1¼ cups water

1. Place the Bai zhu and Chen pi in a non-aluminum saucepan and add the water.

2. Bring the mixture to a boil, then simmer uncovered for at least 20 minutes. Remove from the heat.

3. Strain and drink. Repeat up to 2 times per day. The Take-to-Work Method Afternoon Energy Formula (page 125) includes amounts for a larger batch.

Take-to-Work Method Afternoon Energy Formula

MAKES ABOUT 10 SERVINGS

If you want an energy formula to keep at work, here is a recipe to keep on hand. An ideal setup would be to buy a stainless-steel herb strainer that sits on top of your mug, but you can also use tea bags and fill them as needed.

10 tablespoons Bai zhu (atractylodes)

5 tablespoons Chen pi (tangerine peel)

1. If the herbs have come in pieces larger than a quarter, chop, blend, or grind them into smaller pieces.

2. In a small bowl, thoroughly mix the Bai zhu and Chen pi, then place in an airtight container. Keep the container, a mug, and a tea infuser (or empty tea bags) convenient to your workspace.

3. Infuse 1½ tablespoons of herbs in boiling water for 15 minutes. Strain and drink for afternoon energy.

Decoction for Energy with Reishi

MAKES 3½ CUPS

Ling zhi (reishi) is one of many mushrooms known for their ability to strengthen and give steady, long-term energy. Modern research is showing many other benefits. To dive deeper into the world of medicinal mushrooms used in many of the world's traditional systems of medicine, check out the work of Paul Stamets. He has a TED Talk called "Six Ways Mushrooms Can Save the World," books, and a website with research. The taste is what you would expect a mushroom decoction to taste like. I joke with patients that one way to take herbs like this is to chug it and have a chaser. The taste is part of the medicine, but you also have to be willing and able to drink it daily to receive the benefits.

21 grams Ling zhi (reishi)

4½ cups water

1. Place the Ling zhi in a non-aluminum saucepan and add the water.
2. Bring the mixture to a boil, then simmer uncovered for at least 20 minutes. Remove from the heat.
3. The total amount should be about 3½ cups. Strain and drink by the ½ cup over 7 days.

Frustration

Frustration is a common sign of Liver Qi stagnation and can feel like—or travel alongside—anger. Herbs that regulate or move Qi move us out of a stuck, frustrated pattern so that we can get a better view of what is causing the frustration and try to change the situation around it, so we don't keep returning to these emotions.

Decoction to Free Frustration

MAKES 1 CUP

Xiang fu (cyperus) soothes frustration by freeing stuck Liver Qi. Bai shao (peony) softens and nourishes the Liver Yin, helping Xiang fu ensure a free flow of energy.

3 teaspoons Xiang fu (cyperus)

1 teaspoon Bai shao (peony)

1½ cups water

1. Place the Xiang fu and Bai shao in a non-aluminum saucepan and add the water.

2. Bring the mixture to a boil, then simmer uncovered for 20 minutes. Remove from the heat.

3. Strain and drink.

Infusion to Free Frustration

MAKES 1 CUP

Here is a lighter, flower-based option for pacifying rough emotions. Mei gui hua (rosebud) moves stuck Liver Qi, while He huan pi (albizzia peel) calms the Heart Shen and gently supports the movement of Mei gui hua.

5 or 6 buds Mei gui hua (rosebud)

1 tablespoon He huan pi (albizzia peel)

1½ cups water

1. Place the Mei gui hua and He huan pi in a mug, teapot, or coffee press.

2. Boil the water and pour it over the herbs. Infuse for at least 15 minutes.

3. Strain and drink. Repeat up to 3 times per day.

Gas and Bloating

Gas and bloating are uncomfortable and a sign that digestion is weak and Qi is not circulating properly. If you suffer from chronic gas and bloating, you can incorporate stronger herbs to build and move Qi, like Bai zhu (atractylodes) and Chen pi (tangerine peel). The formula that follows works for immediate relief of gas and bloating.

Decoction for Gas and Bloating

MAKES 1 CUP

Both Xiao hui xiang (fennel) and Yi zhi ren (cardamom) can help ease bloating and gas. If you have coriander seeds in your spice cabinet, you can add a teaspoon of them as well. Drink one or two cups after meals, especially in the afternoon or evening.

3 teaspoons Xiao hui xiang (fennel)

1 teaspoon Yi zhi ren (cardamom) seeds, crushed, or 8 whole pods, crushed

1½ cups water

1. Place the Xiao hui xiang and Yi zhi ren in a non-aluminum saucepan and add the water.
2. Bring the mixture to a boil, then simmer uncovered for 20 minutes. Remove from the heat.
3. Strain and drink. Repeat up to 2 times per day.

Gum Health

In Chinese herbal medicine, the health of the gums is reflective of the health of the Stomach Yin. The Stomach supplies the Yin for the gums. Other digestive symptoms can also be present, including indigestion, heartburn or reflux, gas, diarrhea, or constipation. Avoiding large meals late at night is highly recommended.

Decoction for Healthy Gums

MAKES 7 CUPS

Mai men dong (ophiopogon) nourishes the Stomach Yin, while Ge gen (kudzu) is cool and builds fluids. Jiang huang (turmeric) is also helpful for inflammation, while Da zao (dates) and Yi zhi ren (cardamom) help by adding a little bit of digestive warmth and strength to the other cooling herbs. It takes time to build Yin, so this formula can be used for weeks.

21 grams Mai men dong (ophiopogon)

12 grams Ge gen (kudzu)

12 grams Jiang huang (turmeric)

9 grams Da zao (dates)

3 grams Yi zhi ren (cardamom) seeds or 6 whole pods, crushed

8 cups water

1. Place the Mai men dong, Ge gen, Jiang huang, Da zao, and Yi zhi ren in a non-aluminum stockpot and add the water.

2. Bring the mixture to a boil, then simmer uncovered for 30 minutes. Remove from the heat.

3. Strain into a large, 8-cup glass measuring cup. If the total amount is less than 7 cups, add water to bring it to 7 cups total.

4. Set aside ½ cup as the first dose to drink immediately, then refrigerate the rest.

5. Drink ½ cup morning and evening for 1 week. After 7 days, discard any remaining decoction and make a new batch.

Headaches

Headaches have different causes and underlying patterns. Diagnosis depends on where the pain is located and noticing whether the pain improves with pressure or dislikes pressure and needs stillness.

Decoction for Headache with Dampness

MAKES 1 CUP

A headache that feels like a band around the head includes Dampness as an underlying pattern. It feels more like tightness and pressure than a sharp, stabbing pain. Chuan xiong (ligusticum) is a premiere herb for treating headaches. Here, Du huo (angelica) supports Chuan xiong in dealing with headache pain. Yi yi ren (Job's tears) supports the Dampness-draining effects.

1 tablespoon Chuan xiong (ligusticum)

2 teaspoons Yi yi ren (Job's tears)

2 teaspoons Du huo (angelica)

1½ cups water

1. Place the Chuan xiong, Yi yi ren, and Du huo in a non-aluminum saucepan and add the water.

2. Bring the mixture to a boil, then simmer uncovered for 20 minutes. Remove from the heat.

3. Strain and drink. Repeat up to 3 times per day.

Decoction for Headache with Stagnation

MAKES 1 CUP

The symptoms for this type of headache are pains that are sharp and stabbing and hate pressure; they point to imbalances of Qi or Blood stagnation. Chuan xiong (ligusticum) and Jiang huang (turmeric) treat stagnation and pain, while Ge gen (kudzu) targets pain and tension in the head and shoulders.

1 tablespoon Chuan xiong (ligusticum)

1 teaspoon Jiang huang (turmeric)

1 teaspoon Ge gen (kudzu)

1½ cups water

1. Place the Chuan xiong, Jiang huang, and Ge gen in a non-aluminum saucepan and add the water.

2. Bring the mixture to a boil, then simmer uncovered for 20 minutes. Remove from the heat.

3. Strain and drink. Repeat up to 3 times per day.

Decoction for Headache with Wind

MAKES 1 CUP

A headache at the very top of the head indicates a pattern of disharmony related to the Liver. Migraines are also most often the result of a Liver pattern of disharmony, and both of these can have similar treatment principles and similar herbs in their formulas. Here, Gou teng (cat's claw) anchors the Internal Wind, while Chuan xiong (ligusticum) moves and releases to further help with the pain. If the headache has accompanying Heat symptoms like a sensation of heat or fever and a flushed, red face, add Ju hua (chrysanthemum) to cool. The Decoction for Migraines (page 149) could also be helpful if your migraines are chronic and frequent.

1 tablespoon Chuan xiong (ligusticum)

1½ cups water

2 to 3 teaspoons Gou teng (cat's claw)

2 teaspoons Ju hua (chrysanthemum) (optional)

1. Place the Chuan xiong in a non-aluminum saucepan and add the water.

2. Bring the mixture to a boil, then simmer uncovered for 15 minutes.

3. Add the Gou teng and, if using, the Ju hua and simmer for an additional 5 minutes. Remove from the heat.

4. Strain and drink. Repeat up to 3 times per day.

Decoction for Tension Headache

MAKES 1 CUP

Relaxing the neck and shoulder muscles can help alleviate a tension headache. Ge gen (kudzu) excels at relaxing the shoulders and works with Bai shao (peony) to nourish and relax muscles. He huan pi (albizzia bark) calms and soothes the Shen and gently moves any emotional tension.

3 teaspoons Ge gen (kudzu)

2 teaspoons Bai shao (peony)

2 teaspoons He huan pi (albizzia bark)

1½ cups water

1. Place the Ge gen, Bai shao, and He huan pi in a non-aluminum saucepan and add the water.
2. Bring the mixture to a boil, then simmer uncovered for 20 minutes. Remove from the heat.
3. Strain and drink. Repeat up to 3 times per day.

Heartburn

I was surprised to first learn in a gastroenterology class taught by herbalist David Winston that most heartburn happens from a lack of digestive acids—not an excess of acid. In TCM terminology, this means that the digestion is weak and that the Stomach and Spleen are imbalanced. Antacids help in the short term but don't solve the underlying problem. Some research is beginning to suggest that long-term use of the most common medication for reflux, a proton-pump inhibitor, may increase your risk for gastric cancers.

Decoction for Heartburn

MAKES 1 CUP

For frequent heartburn, try the Decoction for Digestive Strength formula (page 117) earlier in the day, then this formula after meals or in the evening if you suspect you may have heartburn. Mai men dong (ophiopogon) and Ge gen (kudzu) increase the Yin and fluids in the Stomach and are both cooling, while Gui zhi (cinnamon twig) helps warm the digestion and keeps the temperature of the formula from being too cooling.

2 teaspoons Mai men dong (ophiopogon)

2 teaspoons Ge gen (kudzu)

1 teaspoon Gui zhi (cinnamon twig)

1½ cups water

1. Place the Mai men dong, Ge gen, and Gui zhi in a non-aluminum saucepan and add the water.

2. Bring the mixture to a boil, then simmer uncovered for 20 minutes. Remove from the heat.

3. Strain and drink. Repeat up to 3 times per day.

Heart Health

The American Heart Association reports that cardiovascular disease is the leading cause of death in the United States. In addition to diet and lifestyle modification, many Chinese herbs support a healthy cardiovascular system.

Decoction to Promote Heart Health

MAKES 1 CUP

These two herbs are tonic for the cardiovascular system. By building Heart Qi, Ling zhi (reishi) supports Jiang huang (turmeric) in maintaining healthy blood circulation and inhibiting inflammation. You can keep this as a simple herbal decoction for regular use, or you can use it as part of your favorite vegetable or mushroom broth recipe. The website Fungi.com (Fungi Perfecti) has a whole section of mushroom recipes.

2 teaspoons Jiang huang (turmeric)

3 pods Yi zhi ren (cardamom), crushed

1 slice Ling zhi (reishi) (about ¼ inch thick and 2 inches long)

1¼ cups water

1. Place the Jiang huang, Yi zhi ren, and Ling zhi in a non-aluminum saucepan and add the water.
2. Bring the mixture to a boil, then simmer uncovered for 20 minutes. Remove from the heat.
3. Strain and drink. Repeat up to 2 times per day.

Daily Decoction for a Healthy Heart

MAKES 7 CUPS

Traditional usage and modern research both agree the following formula supports heart health. This heart-friendly tonic formula is most effective when taken long-term.

21 grams Sang shen (mulberry)

21 grams Ling zhi (reishi)

12 grams Jiang huang (turmeric)

9 grams Dan shen (salvia)

6 grams Yi zhi ren (cardamom) pods

8 cups water

1. Place the Sang shen, Ling zhi, Jiang huang, Dan shen, and Yi zhi ren in a non-aluminum stockpot and add the water.

2. Bring the mixture to a boil, then simmer uncovered for 30 minutes. Remove from the heat.

3. Strain into a large, 8-cup glass measuring cup. If the total amount is less than 7 cups, add water to bring it to 7 cups total.

4. Set aside ½ cup as the first dose to drink immediately, then refrigerate the rest.

5. Drink ½ cup morning and evening for 1 week. After 7 days, discard any remaining decoction and make a new batch.

PRECAUTIONS: Do not take Dan shen (salvia) if you are on blood-thinning medications.

Cooking Blend for Cardiovascular Health

MAKES 3 TABLESPOONS

This blend includes herbs that support the cardiovascular system. Jiang huang (turmeric) in larger amounts can be a strong flavor. While it easily gives its color to many Indian dishes, it is usually part of a larger blend of multiple spices. When cooking for those new to these flavors, start on the lighter side and increase as they become used to the bold flavors. These are not meant to be overwhelming but background flavors for the dish. As with anything—from practicing yoga to playing an instrument—it is better to get a smaller dose daily than a big dose once a week. This blend can be used in savory and sweet dishes. Making these Chinese herbs a part of your kitchen spice cabinet will keep them handy for regular use while cooking.

Up to 1 tablespoon Gou qi zi (goji berry)

2 or 3 pieces Da zao (dates)

1 to 2 teaspoons Jiang huang (turmeric), grated fresh or powder

1. In a small bowl, mix together the Gou qi zi, Da zao, and Jiang huang.
2. Add to your dish while cooking.

Immunity

In Chinese medicine, the goal is to prevent an illness rather than helping after someone is sick. Many herbs are used to maintain balance and treat the beginnings of disease. In today's language, we refer to them as immune-building herbs or immune tonics. Building immunity and maintaining health require consistency, so these formulas are designed to be used over the long term on a regular basis. Treating any additional patterns of disharmony further benefits immunity.

Cooking Blend for Immunity

MAKES 3 TABLESPOONS

Add this to almost any dish that will be thoroughly heated and cooked for at least 15 minutes, like beans, stews, and soups. Huang qi (astragalus) and Ling zhi (reishi) are both immune tonic herbs. Making these Chinese herbs a part of your kitchen spice cabinet will keep them handy for regular use while cooking.

1 tablespoon Huang qi (astragalus)

1 or 2 slices Ling zhi (reishi) (about 3 to 4 inches long and ¼ inch thick)

1. Add the Huang qi and Ling zhi to your dishes before cooking.

2. When presoaking ingredients like beans or rice, add the herb blend during the soaking process and leave it in for the cooking process.

Decoction for Immunity

MAKES 1 CUP

Huang qi (astragalus) and Ling zhi (reishi) are both classified in Western herbal medicine as adaptogens. This means they help with disease and stress resistance, and this correlates to tonic herbs in Chinese herbal medicine. This formula works best with long-term use.

2 teaspoons Huang qi (astragalus)

1 small slice Ling zhi (reishi)

1¼ cups water

1. Place the Huang qi and Ling zhi in a non-aluminum saucepan and add the water.

2. Bring the mixture to a boil, then simmer uncovered for 20 minutes. Remove from the heat.

3. Strain and drink. Repeat up to 2 times per day.

Jiang huang (Turmeric) Decoction for Immunity

MAKES 1 CUP

Daily, consistent use of turmeric is the most effective way to reap the many health benefits of this herb. If cooking with Jiang huang (turmeric) isn't possible, you can also drink it as a warm drink all by itself or with a little ginger, pepper, or cinnamon for variety. Adding a pinch of pepper or ginger to Jiang huang is an Ayurvedic tradition to increase how well the turmeric is absorbed. A kitchen tip for fresh Jiang huang and ginger is to buy them fresh and freeze them. To use, there's no defrosting necessary; just grate the amount needed and immediately return the rest to the freezer.

1 to 3 teaspoons fresh Jiang huang (turmeric), grated

1 cup water

1. Place the Jiang huang in a mug or teapot.
2. Boil the water and pour over the Jiang huang. Infuse for at least 20 minutes.
3. Strain and drink. For best results, repeat and drink daily.

Incontinence

When dealing with incontinence, there are a few possible underlying patterns. With urination, if you are drinking a healthy amount of water and are well hydrated, your urine should be white to a faint, light yellow color and should be commensurate with intake, meaning you seem to urinate the same amount you drink. Heat makes the urine darker, with less volume, and Cold makes it whiter or lighter, and the volume can seem to be more than you consumed. (Remember that some vitamin supplements can turn your urine artificially yellow.) Heat and Yin deficiency usually make urination more difficult, while Cold and Yang deficiency are the cause of incontinence. This is especially the case if the incontinence started after pregnancy, when many women are depleted in general, or with age.

Decoction for Bladder Support

MAKES 7 CUPS

This formula is very warming, so if there is also some Blood and Yin deficiency, you can balance it by following the natural flow of Yin and Yang. Take this warming, Yang formula in the morning, when Yang is naturally increasing to give a lift to Qi for the day. Then use a cooler, Yin formula like the Decoction for Deeper Sleep (page 144) to help at night, when Yin should be dominant and rest and sleep are needed.

25 grams Huang qi
(astragalus)

21 grams Bai zhu
(atractylodes)

15 grams Xu duan (teasel)

12 grams Da zao (dates)

12 grams Shan zhu yu
(cornus)

8 cups water

1. Place the Huang qi, Bai zhu, Xu duan, Da zao, and Shan zhu yu in a non-aluminum stockpot and add the water.

2. Bring the mixture to a boil, then simmer uncovered for 30 minutes. Remove from the heat.

3. Strain into a large, 8-cup glass measuring cup. If the total amount is less than 7 cups, add water to bring it to 7 cups total.

4. Set aside ½ cup as the first dose to drink immediately, then refrigerate the rest.

5. Drink ½ cup morning and evening for 1 week. After 7 days, discard any remaining decoction and make a new batch.

Insomnia

In Chinese medicine, there is a diagnostic difference between having trouble *falling* asleep and having trouble *staying* asleep. The first is Blood deficiency, the second Yin deficiency. Stagnation can also be a factor, so sleep formulas often contain herbs that help smooth the flow of Qi. In practice, I've seen insomnia resolve quickly but also cases with multiple patterns that take longer to untangle.

Infusion for Falling Asleep

MAKES 1 CUP

He huan hua (albizzia flower) helps calm the Shen to prepare for falling asleep. Long yan rou (longan berry) assists He huan hua in calming Shen and building Blood. Together, they help with overthinking and worrying so they do not keep you from drifting off to sleep. Add this formula to a nightly sleep routine to maximize its effectiveness.

3 tablespoons He huan hua (albizzia flower)

2 tablespoons Long yan rou (longan berry)

1 cup water

1. Place the He huan hua and Long yan rou in a large mug.

2. Boil the water and pour it over the herbs. Cover and steep for 15 to 20 minutes.

3. Strain and drink up to 2 times in the evening. If one cup a half hour before bedtime doesn't help, add a second cup between dinner and bedtime. If you like, you can also eat the Long yan rou after they've steeped.

Decoction for Deeper Sleep

MAKES 7 CUPS

When the problem isn't falling asleep but waking up one or more times at night, more Yin is needed to stay resting deeply. It takes a while to build Yin reserves, so this is a formula to use consistently to nourish Yin and improve sleep.

24 grams Tian men dong (asparagus root)

18 grams Bai shao (peony)

18 grams He huan pi (albizzia peel)

9 grams Dan shen (salvia)

9 grams Da zao (dates)

8 cups water

1. Place the Tian men dong, Bai shao, He huan pi, Dan shen, and Da zao in a non-aluminum stockpot and add the water.

2. Bring the mixture to a boil, then simmer uncovered for 30 minutes. Remove from the heat.

3. Strain into a large, 8-cup glass measuring cup. If the total amount is less than 7 cups, add water to bring it to 7 cups total.

4. Set aside ½ cup as the first dose to drink immediately, then refrigerate the rest.

5. Drink ½ cup after lunch (or in the afternoon) and ½ cup a half hour before bed for 1 week. After 7 days, discard any remaining decoction and make a new batch.

Decoction to Calm the Mind at Bedtime

MAKES 2 CUPS

This can be used alone or added on to one of the other insomnia formulas. Long yan rou (longan berry) is excellent for helping relax excessive thinking, and He huan pi (albizzia peel) calms the Shen and gently moves the Qi to help pacify the Liver. If you find Long yan rou in season and fresh (check your local Asian grocers), you can eat it fresh instead of making this decoction.

3 tablespoons Long yan rou (longan)

1 teaspoon He huan pi (albizzia peel)

2 teaspoons Ling zhi (reishi)

2½ cups water

1. Place the Long yan rou, He huan pi, and Ling zhi in a non-aluminum saucepan and add the water.

2. Bring the mixture to a boil, then simmer uncovered for 30 minutes. Remove from the heat.

3. Strain and drink before bedtime. With insomnia it can be helpful to have multiple doses in the hours before bed. Ideally with this formula you would drink one cup 2 hours before bed and then the second cup an hour before sleeping.

Menstrual Issues

Women tolerate pain, discomfort, and inconvenience around menstruation, much of it unnecessary. A "normal" period should have only minor cramping and discomfort, and the period should occur regularly every 28 to 32 days. Bleeding should last three to six days and should not be excessive. Chinese herbal medicine can help make menstruation a far less disruptive event every month.

Herbal Oil for Menstrual Cramps

MAKES ONE 16-OUNCE JAR

This oil moves Qi and Blood with Xiang fu (cyperus) and Jiang huang (turmeric), circulates and calms spasms with Gui zhi (cinnamon twig), drains Dampness with Yi yi ren (Job's tears), and nourishes Liver Blood and Yin with Bai shao (peony). To make it even more relaxing and soothing, warm the oil before applying. Place the jar of oil in hot water or use a double boiler. The Ayurvedic retreat center where I first experienced Abhyanga, a type of warm oil massage, used small slow cookers to warm the oil gently without overheating it. You could also soak gauze or thin cloth in the oil to place over the lower abdomen. Anything with Jiang huang takes on its beautiful orange color, so this oil may temporarily stain your skin or permanently discolor clothing.

2 tablespoons Xiang fu (cyperus)

2 tablespoons Jiang huang (turmeric)

2 tablespoons Yi yi ren (Job's tears)

2 tablespoons Bai shao (peony)

1 tablespoon Gui zhi (cinnamon twig)

Oil of your choice (sesame, coconut)

1. Fill a 16-ounce jar with the Xiang fu, Jiang huang, Yi yi ren, Bai shao, and Gui zhi, leaving space between the top of the herbs and the top of the jar.

2. Cover completely with the oil and secure the lid. It is important that the herbs are completely covered and none are above the oil, as this can ruin the oil.

3. Let the oil sit for 6 weeks, then strain and store in a glass container. Refrigerate and keep for 6 months to a year.

4. Use 1 to 3 tablespoons for abdominal massage, preferably warm. A cloth soaked in oil can also be placed across the abdomen.

Decoction for Menstrual Cramps

MAKES 1 CUP

The TCM diagnosis for menstrual cramping is stagnation, either of Qi or Blood or both. These two herbs excel at stopping menstrual cramps. Chuan xiong (ligusticum) moves the Blood, and Xiang fu (cyperus) moves the Qi.

2 teaspoons Chuan xiong (ligusticum)

2 teaspoons Xiang fu (cyperus)

1¼ cups water

1. Place the Chuan xiong and Xiang fu in a non-aluminum saucepan and add the water.

2. Bring the mixture to a boil, then simmer uncovered for 20 minutes. Remove from the heat.

3. Strain and drink. Repeat up to 2 times per day.

4. Use 1 to 3 tablespoons for abdominal massage, preferably warm. A cloth soaked in oil can also be placed across the abdomen.

Decoction for Menstrual Cramps with Blood Deficiency

MAKES 2 CUPS

Menstrual cramps and other pains are symptoms of stuck Qi that isn't moving the way it should be. Smoothing and moving Liver Qi goes a long way in eliminating cramps. Xiang fu (cyperus) is used frequently with menstrual issues for its ability to move stuck Qi, while Bai shao (peony) soothes the Liver Yin and Blood. Jiang huang (turmeric) helps with the pain by promoting movement, as well. This is not a long-term formula: Take it only when cramps are present.

1 tablespoon Xiang fu (cyperus)

1 tablespoon Bai shao (peony)

1 teaspoon Jiang huang (turmeric)

2½ cups water

1. Place the Xiang fu, Bai shao, and Jiang huang in a non-aluminum saucepan and add the water.

2. Bring the mixture to a boil, then simmer uncovered for 20 minutes. Remove from the heat.

3. Strain and drink over the next hour. Repeat if cramps continue, but no more than 3 times in 1 day.

Migraines

Migraines can have various triggers and causes, but in TCM, one of the patterns underlying them is Internal Wind. Internal Wind involves the Liver in some way, whether it is Liver Yin deficiency, Heat, or Liver Wind.

Decoction for Migraines (Based on Tian Ma Gou Teng Yin)

MAKES 7 CUPS

Migraines are painful and can be a massive interruption to daily life. This formula is designed to help migraines and prevent them by anchoring Wind and building Yin and Blood to prevent Wind. In Chinese herbal medicine, a formula for Wind and migraines is taken regularly and preventively, not just when a migraine starts. Gou teng (cat's claw) anchors Wind, while Tian men dong (asparagus root) and Bai shao (peony) nourish Kidney and Liver Yin. Da zao (dates) is included to help with digestion and to keep the other ingredients from being too cold. Pulling from our beginner apothecary of 35 single herbs, this formula takes its lead from Tian Ma Gou Teng Yin, the archetypal formula to treat Liver Wind.

12 grams Bai shao (peony)

9 grams Xu duan (teasel)

9 grams Da zao (dates)

6 grams Tian men dong (asparagus root)

8 cups water

21 grams Gou teng (cat's claw)

6 grams Ju hua (chrysanthemum)

1. Place the Bai shao, Xu duan, Da zao, and Tian men dong in a non-aluminum stockpot and add the water.

2. Bring the mixture to a boil, then simmer uncovered for 25 minutes. Remove from the heat.

3. Add the Gou teng and Ju hua and simmer for another 5 minutes.

4. Strain into a large, 8-cup glass measuring cup. If the total amount is less than 7 cups, add water to bring it to 7 cups total.

5. Set aside ½ cup as the first dose to drink immediately, then refrigerate the rest.

6. Drink ½ cup morning and evening for 1 week. After 7 days, discard any remaining decoction and make a new batch.

Muscle Cramps

Leg cramps, especially the calf cramps sometimes called charley horses, are uncomfortable, can wake you up in the middle of the night, and can be severe enough that they leave muscles sore for hours after. One of the primary patterns underlying muscle cramps is Blood deficiency.

Decoction for Preventing Leg and Muscle Cramps

MAKES 7 CUPS

Bai shao (peony) is *the* herb for muscle cramps, pain, and spasms, which are most often due to Liver Blood or Yin deficiency. Da zao (dates) is added to help build the Qi and Blood and to balance the coolness of Mei gui hua (rosebud) and Bai shao. The smaller amount of Mei gui hua ensures the Qi is circulating properly.

30 grams Bai shao (peony)

15 grams Da zao (dates)

8 cups water

6 grams Mei gui hua (rosebud)

1. Place the Bai shao and Da zao in a non-aluminum stockpot and add the water.

2. Bring the mixture to a boil, then simmer uncovered for 30 minutes. Remove from the heat.

3. Add the Mei gui hua and infuse for 5 minutes.

4. Strain into a large, 8-cup glass measuring cup. If the total amount is less than 7 cups, add water to bring it to 7 cups total.

5. Set aside ½ cup as the first dose to drink immediately, then refrigerate the rest.

6. Drink ½ cup morning and evening for 1 week. After 7 days, discard any remaining decoction and make a new batch.

Compress for Muscle Cramps

MAKES ENOUGH FOR 5 DAYS

The Spleen is in charge of the muscles. With this formula you combine the Spleen Qi tonics of Huang qi (astragalus) and Da zao (dates) to support them. Bai shao (peony) is a powerful herb for relaxing muscles, ligaments, and tendons and easing cramps by nourishing Liver Blood and Yin. Jiang huang (turmeric) moves any stagnation, and Ge gen (kudzu) is moistening and relaxing, especially for the upper body. The temperature of this formula is fairly balanced between cool and warm herbs.

½ cup Bai shao (peony)

½ cup Jiang huang (turmeric)

½ cup Ge gen (kudzu)

¼ cup Huang qi (astragalus)

¼ cup Da zao (dates)

8 cups water

Clean, dry cloth

1. Place the Bai shao, Jiang huang, Ge gen, Huang qi, and Da zao in a non-aluminum stockpot and add the water.

2. Bring the mixture to a boil, then simmer uncovered for 25 minutes.

3. Strain into a large, 8-cup glass measuring cup.

4. Wash the area to be soaked, soak the cloth in the warm herbal decoction, and apply to the area for 15 to 30 minutes.

5. Store this decoction in the refrigerator and use again for up to 5 days. The decoction should be warmed before applying to a compress. Hot water can be added, or the decoction can be heated in the microwave. Use caution not to burn the skin.

PRECAUTIONS: Jiang huang (turmeric) will discolor or stain skin and clothing.

Compress for Muscle Cramps with Heat

MAKES ENOUGH FOR 5 DAYS

If your pain and cramping are accompanied by Heat, or the pain feels worse or doesn't like Heat, then Mu dan pi (tree peony) can be added to the Compress for Muscle Cramps formula (page 151). This enhances the formula's heat-clearing properties.

¼ cup Bai shao (peony)

¼ cup Huang qi (astragalus)

¼ cup Da zao (dates)

½ cup Jiang huang (turmeric)

¼ cup Mu dan pi (tree peony)

½ cup Ge gen (kudzu)

8 cups water

Clean, dry cloth

1. Place the Bai shao, Huang qi, Da zao, Jiang huang, Mu dan pi, and Ge gen in a non-aluminum stockpot and add the water.

2. Bring the mixture to a boil, then simmer uncovered for 25 minutes.

3. Strain into a large, 8-cup glass measuring cup.

4. Wash the area to be soaked, soak the cloth in the warm herbal decoction, and apply to the area for 15 to 30 minutes.

5. Store this decoction in the refrigerator and use again for up to 5 days. The decoction should be warmed before applying to a compress. Hot water can be added, or the decoction can be heated in the microwave. Use caution not to burn the skin.

Neck and Shoulder Pain

Chinese herbal medicine recognizes that some herbs have a direction or affinity for a specific part of the body. Some herbs have a downward action; some have a lifting action. Some herbs have the ability to guide the rest of the formula into an area, like the upper or lower body. These herbs work in the formula with other herbs to correct imbalances like stagnation.

Decoction for Relief of Neck and Shoulder Pain

MAKES 7 CUPS

Ge gen (kudzu) gives this formula direction and attention to the shoulders and upper body, while Gui zhi (cinnamon twig) circulates and warms. Dan shen (salvia) helps Gui zhi with circulation, but with a balancing coolness. Blood deficiency can be accompanied by low-grade, persistent tension and inability to relax. Bai shao (peony) relaxes and nourishes sinews, ligaments, and tendons by building Blood.

21 grams Ge gen (kudzu)

21 grams Bai shao (peony)

15 grams Du huo (angelica)

6 grams Dan shen (salvia)

8 cups water

12 grams Gui zhi
    (cinnamon twig)

1. Place the Ge gen, Bai shao, Du huo, and Dan shen in a non-aluminum stockpot and add the water.

2. Bring the mixture to a boil, then simmer uncovered for 25 minutes.

3. Add the Gui zhi and simmer for another 5 minutes. Remove from the heat.

4. Strain into a large, 8-cup glass measuring cup. If the total amount is less than 7 cups, add water to bring it to 7 cups total.

5. Set aside ½ cup as the first dose to drink immediately, then refrigerate the rest.

6. Drink ½ cup morning and evening for 1 week. After 7 days, discard any remaining decoction and make a new batch.

Herbal Oil for Neck and Shoulder Pain

MAKES ONE 16-OUNCE JAR

Much as in the internal formula, Ge gen (kudzu) relaxes the upper body, while Du huo (angelica) and Gui zhi (cinnamon twig) help warm and ease pain. Bai shao (peony) builds Blood to nourish and relax the muscles.

2 tablespoons Ge gen (kudzu)

2 tablespoons Bai shao (peony)

2 tablespoons Du huo (angelica)

2 teaspoons Gui zhi (cinnamon twig)

14 ounces oil of your choice

1. Fill a 16-ounce glass container with the Ge gen, Bai shao, Du huo, and Gui zhi, leaving space between the top of the herbs and the top of the jar.

2. Cover the herbs completely with the oil and secure the lid. (It is important that no herbs are above the oil and remain uncovered, as this can ruin the oil.)

3. Let the oil sit for 6 weeks, then strain and store in a glass container. Store in the refrigerator. The oil will keep for 6 months to a year.

4. Use 1 to 3 tablespoons oil, and massage into the shoulders, neck, and upper back.

Pediatrics

Herbal medicine can be helpful for children, but kids can be resistant to new tastes. Tub teas are an excellent answer, with the child soaking in a tub full of helpful herbs. (These remedies are also useful for adults who are resistant to ingesting herbs!) I have used these with children of all ages; however, due to varying skin sensitivity, always test smaller areas and supervise children when using. For children under the age of two, consult a Chinese herbalist before using.

Calming Tub Tea

MAKES ENOUGH FOR 3 BATHS

This tub tea is ideal for soothing little ones in preparation for bedtime. Store your formula in an airtight container and use within a month, since ground herbs lose potency faster. You can add one cup of Epsom salt to the mix if you wish. Epsom salt contains magnesium, which helps relax the muscles. It is helpful for tension, aches, and pains as well as relieving itchy skin. A popular and overall safe additive to baths, it is possible to get too much of this good thing, so use in moderation. For babies and toddlers, you can always check with your pediatrician before using to make sure they are right for your child.

1 cup Bai shao (peony)

1 cup He huan pi or He huan hua (albizzia)

1 cup Mei gui hua (rosebud)

1 cup Epsom salt (optional)

1. Grind the Bai shao and He huan pi (if using the bark), then combine with the Mei gui hua and He huan hua (if using the flower).

2. Mix in a container with a lid, adding the Epsom salt if you choose.

3. At bath time, place 1 cup of well-mixed blend into a thin cotton sock, or place in the center of a tea towel and tightly close with a rubber band or string. Place in the warm bath water, squeezing the tub tea to help infuse the herbs into the water.

Warming Tub Tea

MAKES ENOUGH FOR 2 BATHS

Make sure to use this warming tub tea within a week or two, as the Gui zhi (cinnamon twig) will lose its beneficial oils. Feel free to add ¼ cup Epsom salt to the mix. This is excellent for the cold winter months and cold and flu season.

1 cup Gui zhi
   (cinnamon twig)

1 cup Xiao hui xiang
   (fennel)

¼ cup Epsom salt (optional)

1. Grind the Gui zhi and Xiao hui xiang and mix in a container with a lid, adding the Epsom salt if you choose.

2. At bath time, place 1 cup of well-mixed blend into a thin cotton sock, or place in the center of a tea towel and tightly close with a rubber band or string. Place in the warm bath water, squeezing the tub tea to help infuse the herbs into the water.

Skin-Soothing Tub Tea

MAKES ENOUGH FOR 2 BATHS

Ju hua (chrysanthemum) and Mei gui hua (rosebud) are calming and cooling for red, irritated skin conditions. Adding oatmeal helps if there is dryness. This tub tea is great for soothing rashes, eczema, sunburn, and itchy bug bites.

1 cup Ju hua (chrysanthemum)

1 cup Mei gui hua (rosebud)

1 cup oatmeal (instant is best) (optional)

1. Grind the Ju hua and Mei gui hua and mix in a container with a lid, adding the oatmeal if you choose.

2. At bath time, place 1 cup of well-mixed blend into a thin cotton sock, or place in the center of a tea towel and tightly close with a rubber band or string. Place in the warm bath water, squeezing and soaking the tub tea to help infuse the herbs into the water.

Digestive Help Tub Tea

MAKES ENOUGH FOR 2 OR 3 BATHS

Huang qi (astragalus) is a warming Qi tonic that helps digestion. Shan zha (hawthorn) helps with slow digestion, while Da zao (dates) supports Huang qi in building Spleen Qi to improve digestion.

1 cup Huang qi (astragalus)

1 cup Shan zha (hawthorn)

½ cup Da zao (dates)

1 cup Epsom salt (optional)

1. Grind the Huang qi, Shan zha, and Da zao and mix in a container with a lid, adding the Epsom salt if you choose.

2. At bath time, place 1 cup of well-mixed blend into a thin cotton sock, or place in the center of a tea towel and tightly close with a rubber band or string. Place in the warm bath water, squeezing and soaking the tub tea to help infuse the herbs into the water.

Digestive Decoction for Children

MAKES 1 CUP

Children can drink this in the morning and evening. How they drink it depends on their taste tolerance. Some children prefer a dropperful farther back in their mouth to bypass some taste buds. Some prefer to water it down and sip it more slowly. My favorite method of dilution for pediatric herbal formulas is unsweetened fruit teas. Children can experience frequent, mild Spleen Qi deficiency that leads to upset tummies, loose stools, excess mucus, and head congestion especially after eating. Some kinds of constipation can also be helped with this formula as well, due to the moistening nature of Da zao (dates) and the moving qualities of Chen pi (tangerine peel).

1 tablespoon Bai zhu (atractylodes)

3 or 4 pieces Da zao (dates)

2 teaspoons Chen pi (tangerine peel)

4 or 5 pieces Shan zha (hawthorn)

1½ cups water

1. Place the Bai zhu, Da zao, Chen pi, and Shan zha in a non-aluminum saucepan and add the water.

2. Bring the mixture to a boil, then simmer gently, uncovered, for 20 minutes. Remove from the heat.

3. Strain and store in a covered glass container. Refrigerate, but add to warm water or warm unsweetened fruit tea like Celestial Seasonings peach or blueberry flavor before giving to your child. Children can take 1 to 3 tablespoons of this decoction at a time.

Warming Digestive Decoction for Children

MAKES 1 CUP

Refrigerator syndrome is a term used for when anyone—but especially children—eats a lot of cold foods and foods straight from the refrigerator, like cereal, yogurts, juices, and fruits. This cold temperature weakens digestion and can lead to increased mucus production. Allowing foods to warm to room temperature and eating cooked foods help, as well as taking warming herbs to strengthen digestion. Children can drink this in the morning and evening. How they drink it depends on their taste tolerance. My favorite method of dilution for pediatric herbal formulas is unsweetened fruit teas.

2 teaspoons Xiao hui xiang (fennel)

2 pods Yi zhi ren (cardamom), crushed

4 pieces Da zao (dates)

1½ cups water

1. Place the Xiao hui xiang, Yi zhi ren, and Da zao in a non-aluminum saucepan and add the water.

2. Bring the mixture to a boil, then simmer gently, uncovered, for 20 minutes. Remove from the heat.

3. Strain and store in a covered glass container. Refrigerate, but add to warm water or warm unsweetened fruit tea like Celestial Seasonings peach or blueberry flavor before giving to your child. Children can take 1 to 3 tablespoons of this decoction at a time.

Sleep Decoction for Children

MAKES 1 CUP

Children can drink this in the morning and evening. This formula is a calming, relaxing blend that helps settle the emotions. This can be used at bedtime to help children fall asleep faster or to help with disturbed sleep and waking up during the night. It is not heavily sedating but soothing, so it is excellent for use before or during travel.

1 tablespoon He huan hua (albizzia flower)

4 or 5 buds Mei gui hua (rosebud)

6 or 7 pieces Long yan rou (longan berry)

1½ cups water

1. Place the He huan hua, Mei gui hua, and Long yan rou in a non-aluminum saucepan and add the water.

2. Bring the mixture to a boil, then simmer gently, uncovered, for 20 minutes. Remove from the heat.

3. Strain and store in a covered glass container. Refrigerate, but add to warm water or warm unsweetened fruit tea like Celestial Seasonings peach or blueberry flavor before giving to your child. Children can take 1 to 3 tablespoons of this decoction at a time.

Postpartum

Pregnancy and childbirth use a lot of Qi and Blood, with the demands of caring for a newborn further depleting reserves. All parents need support, but parents who have recently given birth need extra support due to the many physical demands of pregnancy and childbirth. Postpartum support also applies to people who have miscarried, and Chinese herbal medicine can support them as well.

Postpartum Syrup

MAKES ABOUT 16 OUNCES

This syrup is based on the formula Ba zhen tang (Eight Treasures Decoction), which contains eight herbs to build both Qi and Blood. Here, a syrup is helpful, because families with new babies are often tired and too busy to make herbal decoctions. Syrups can be made before the baby arrives and stored or given as a present to new parents. This formula can be taken for months to help strengthen not only the birth parent but any parent who is lacking sleep and needs support.

½ cup Da zao (dates)

½ cup Gou qi zi (goji berry)

30 grams Bai zhu (atractylodes)

30 grams Bai shao (peony)

15 grams Fu ling (poria)

15 grams Tian men dong (asparagus root)

12 grams Huang qi (astragalus)

8 cups water

12 grams Chen pi (tangerine peel)

1. Place the Da zao, Gou qi zi, Bai zhu, Bai shao, Fu ling, Tian men dong, and Huang qi in a large, non-aluminum stockpot and add the water.

2. Bring the mixture to a boil, then simmer for 30 minutes. Add the Chen pi and continue simmering until the liquid is thick, stirring occasionally. After 45 minutes, check the thickness of the liquid (this can be cooked for up to 60 minutes). When the liquid begins to look syrupy, remove from the heat and cool.

3. Before straining the mixture, use a blender, food processor, or potato masher to smash up the fruits and herbs to extract all of the rich juices and liquid from them.

2 tablespoons water, ghee, or coconut oil

1 teaspoon Xiao hui xiang (fennel)

1 teaspoon Rou gui (cinnamon bark)

8 pods Yi zhi ren (cardamom), crushed

Molasses

4. Using a large, fine-mesh strainer, press out the mixture into a large, 8-cup glass measuring cup. If the mixture is thick, use a spoon or spatula to help press it through the strainer.

5. Make a note of how much syrupy decoction is in the measuring cup. You will be measuring out the same amount of molasses for a 1:1 ratio to make the syrup (it takes that much sugar to preserve the decoction).

6. Into the now-empty stockpot, place the water, ghee, or coconut oil and add the Xiao hui xiang, Rou gui, and Yi zhi ren. Simmer for 1 to 2 minutes, then add the syrupy decoction back to the stockpot and stir to combine. Add equal parts molasses and stir to blend completely. Continue to stir and cook on low heat for 10 minutes, then remove from the heat.

7. Syrups are best stored in a glass container like a mason jar. Refrigerate and use within 6 months to a year.

8. Take 1 to 2 tablespoons per day, with warm water or in food like a smoothie or oatmeal.

Postpartum Decoction

MAKES 7 CUPS

If there are reasons to prefer a decoction to a making a syrup, like blood-sugar levels, you can use this formula instead of the Postpartum Syrup on page 162. New parents can be overwhelmed and sleep deprived, so I do not normally recommend decoctions for new parents, as they take more energy to prepare. For this formula, I emphasize the slow-cooker instructions for ease of cooking, but it is also helpful if a family member or friend can cook the decoction for the parent who has given birth. Partners and parents who have not given birth can try one of the Qi tonifying energy formulas (starting on page 123) to support them in this time, as they may not need the significant nourishing of Blood and Yin that you find in the postpartum formulas.

24 grams Bai zhu (atractylodes)

24 grams Bai shao (peony)

15 grams Long yan rou (longan)

12 grams Fu ling (poria)

12 grams Da zao (dates)

12 grams Tian men dong (asparagus root)

6 grams Chen pi (tangerine peel)

6 pods Yi zhi ren (cardamom), crushed

8 cups water

1. Place the Bai zhu, Bai shao, Long yan rou, Fu ling, Da zao, Tian men dong, Chen pi, and Yi zhi ren in the slow cooker and add the water. Decoct the herbs on the lowest setting for about 8 hours or overnight. Check periodically to see whether more water is needed to cover the herbs completely. When the cooking is complete, turn off the slow cooker and allow the mixture to cool.

2. Strain the mixture over a large, 8-cup measuring cup, and pour the liquid into a bowl, leaving the herbs in the strainer. This is the herbal decoction you will drink.

3. Refrigerate the liquid and discard the cooked herbs. Seven cups of decocted herbs lasts a week and divides evenly into a dose of ½ cup twice a day. If you end up with more, divide what you have by 7 and drink it over the week. If you end up with less, add water to bring the total to 7 cups. (This is an inexact science because different dried herbs absorb different amounts of water during the cooking process.) After 7 days, discard any remaining decoction and prepare the next week's herbal formula.

Premenstrual Stress

In the language of TCM patterns, premenstrual syndrome (PMS) is due to a disharmony between the Liver and the Spleen. The Liver and the Spleen can be like siblings in a fight, with the Liver bullying the Spleen and upsetting the rest of the family. The Spleen has trouble doing its work because it has been bullied.

Decoction to Harmonize the Liver and Spleen

MAKES 7 CUPS

Here, Bai zhu (atractylodes) tonifies the Spleen Qi, with Bai shao (peony) building Liver Blood and Xiang fu (cyperus) smoothing out stuck Liver Qi. This formula works best when you take it the week before your menstrual period starts. You can continue taking it throughout the cycle. It helps with cramps, aches and pains, fatigue, and emotional upset or frustration.

24 grams Bai zhu (atractylodes)

24 grams Bai shao (peony)

15 grams Xiang fu (cyperus)

8 cups water

1. Place the Bai zhu, Bai shao, and Xiang fu in a non-aluminum stockpot and add the water.

2. Bring the mixture to a boil, then simmer for 30 minutes.

3. Strain into a large, 8-cup glass measuring cup. If the total amount is less than 7 cups, add water to bring it to 7 cups total.

4. Set aside ½ cup as the first dose to drink immediately, then refrigerate the rest.

5. Drink ½ cup morning and evening for 1 week. After 7 days, discard any remaining decoction and make a new batch.

Decoction for PMS with Menstrual Cramps

MAKES 7 CUPS

When PMS always includes cramping, especially persistent, strong cramping, add Chuan xiong (ligusticum) to strengthen the soothing actions of the Decoction to Harmonize the Liver and Spleen (page 165).

9 grams Chuan xiong (ligusticum)

24 grams Bai zhu (atractylodes)

24 grams Bai shao (peony)

15 grams Xiang fu (cyperus)

8 cups water

1. Place the Chuan xiong, Bai zhu, Bai shao, and Xiang fu in a non-aluminum stockpot and add the water.

2. Bring the mixture to a boil, then simmer for 30 minutes.

3. Strain into a large, 8-cup glass measuring cup. If the total amount is less than 7 cups, add water to bring it to 7 cups total.

4. Set aside ½ cup as the first dose to drink immediately, then refrigerate the rest.

5. Drink ½ cup morning and evening for 1 week. After 7 days, discard any remaining decoction and make a new batch.

Decoction to Harmonize with Bloating and Edema

MAKES 7 CUPS

When the Liver bullies the Spleen and it stops managing fluids properly, bloating and edema can be a part of PMS. Fu ling (poria) drains Dampness and can help with the water weight gain, bloating, and edema that occur during the menstrual cycle.

12 grams Fu ling (poria)

24 grams Bai zhu (atractylodes)

24 grams Bai shao (peony)

15 grams Xiang fu (cyperus)

8 cups water

1. Place the Fu ling, Bai zhu, Bai shao, and Xiang fu in a non-aluminum stockpot and add the water.

2. Bring the mixture to a boil, then simmer for 30 minutes.

3. Strain into a large, 8-cup glass measuring cup. If the total amount is less than 7 cups, add water to bring it to 7 cups total.

4. Set aside ½ cup as the first dose to drink immediately, then refrigerate the rest.

5. Drink ½ cup morning and evening for 1 week. After 7 days, discard any remaining decoction and make a new batch.

Sinus Infections

Many Chinese herbs that treat the Lungs and colds help with the nose and sinus issues. Sinus infections range from uncomfortable to painful, can trigger headaches, and can linger and be a challenge to treat.

Decoction for Sinus Infections

MAKES 1 CUP

Green cardamom extracts have been used to fight sinus infections and performed so well that researchers recommend cardamom as a first line of defense. Here Jiang huang (turmeric) is added as another herb that helps with colds, infections, and inflammation. If your sinus infection has occurred along with a cold or allergies, add this to one of the cold formulas if that is appropriate. There are a lot of options for turmeric out there, from fresh in the grocery store to dried or powdered. If you buy it fresh from the grocery store, it can go bad before you can use it all, so a trick is to freeze it and grate what you need from the frozen root. For a sinus infection, it is a good idea to take this formula multiple times per day for at least four days.

2 teaspoons Yi zhi ren (cardamom) seeds or 10 to 12 whole pods, crushed

2 teaspoons fresh Jiang huang (turmeric)

1½ cups water

1. Place the Yi zhi ren and Jiang huang into a non-aluminum cooking pot and add the water.

2. Bring the mixture to a boil, then simmer uncovered for 20 minutes. Remove from the heat.

3. Strain the decoction and drink over the next 30 minutes. Repeat up to 3 times a day.

Skin Health

Red, irritated skin can be annoying, painful, and, for some, embarrassing. Chinese herbs can cool the Heat and soothe the irritation topically.

Facial Steam with Mei gui hua

MAKES 4 CUPS

Mei gui hua (rosebud) is good for the complexion and can be used for less serious medicinal herbal preparations like this relaxing facial steam. Excellent for astringing and cooling the skin, Mei gui hua is ideal for soothing red, irritated skin. It smells nice and works well. This is a treat and a chance to play with herbs in fun ways.

5 to 8 buds Mei gui hua (rosebud), crushed

4 cups boiling water

Bowl and clean, dry towel

1. In a large bowl, place the Mei gui hua and add the boiling water.
2. Infuse the Mei gui hua for a few minutes.
3. When the water begins to cool to a safe temperature, lower your face (or any red, irritated skin) to catch the steam coming from the bowl. Use a towel to help aim the steam, or put it over your head to keep the steam close.

Sprains and Bruises

The martial arts developed over centuries alongside Chinese medicine, so naturally there are herbal solutions for injuries, accidents, and accompanying pain.

Compress for Pain from Injury

MAKES ENOUGH FOR 5 DAYS

This compress is for application on an injury, sprain, bruise, or area of pain. The pain could be sharp and stabbing and in the same spot, like the inflammation in runner's knee or a twisted ankle. Jiang huang (turmeric) and Chuan xiong (ligusticum) reduce inflammation and move Blood stagnation that causes pain. Both are warming and are balanced by the coolness of the Qi-moving Mei gui hua (rosebud). Bai shao (peony) relaxes and nourishes the ligaments, tendons, and muscles through its Liver Blood and Yin tonic properties.

½ cup Jiang huang (turmeric), grated or diced

½ cup Chuan xiong (ligusticum)

½ cup Mei gui hua (rosebud)

½ cup Bai shao (peony)

8 cups water

Clean, dry cloth

1. Place the Jiang huang, Chuan xiong, Mei gui hua, and Bai shao in a non-aluminum cooking pot and add the water.

2. Bring the mixture to a boil, then simmer for 25 minutes.

3. Strain into a large, 8-cup glass measuring cup.

4. Wash the area to be soaked, soak the cloth in the warm herbal decoction, and apply to the area for 15 to 30 minutes.

5. Store this decoction in the refrigerator and use again for up to 5 days. To warm the decoction before use on subsequent days, you can add boiling water or microwave the decoction. You want the compress to be warm to very warm; test the temperature to ensure it is not too hot and will not burn the skin.

PRECAUTIONS: Jiang huang can stain clothing and skin.

Summer Heat

The long, sunny days of summer are full of fun, but excessive sun exposure and heat can lead to what Chinese medicine terms *summer heat*. Symptoms include irritability, thirst, fatigue, and feeling overheated and can encompass Western terms like *heat exhaustion* and *heat stroke*. The herbs in the following formulas alleviate thirst, cool, and dissipate heat so you feel refreshed. A fun fact: Watermelon has a Pinyin name—Xi gua—and is included in the category of Clearing Summer Heat. A favorite summer fruit is also medicinal!

Summer Cooler

MAKES 8 CUPS

Ju hua (chrysanthemum) makes a refreshing summer drink. While this formula technically makes 8 cups, this is meant to be enjoyed for its taste, so you can make it stronger or weaker based on your personal preference. It can also be the basis for fun summer recipes made by adding other types of tea, from green and white teas to unsweetened fruit teas like hibiscus or peach.

¼ cup Ju hua (chrysanthemum)

4 cups hot water

4 cups cold water

1. In a large glass container like an 8-cup measuring cup, place the Ju hua and add the hot water.

2. Infuse, covering if possible, for at least 15 minutes. If you are adding other teas, include them in the infusion.

3. Once the herbs have infused, strain out the herbs and add the cold water. Enjoy liberally.

Summer Cooler 2

MAKES 8 CUPS

Ju hua (chrysanthemum) is cooling, while Da zao (dates) nourishes the Spleen and Stomach. Gou qi zi (goji berry) adds Yin and flavor. The Da zao and Gou qi zi add stronger, sweeter flavors to the Ju hua, and the Gou qi zi adds a beautiful red hue to the drink.

¼ cup Ju hua (chrysanthemum)

1 to 3 Da zao (dates)

1 to 2 tablespoons Gou qi zi (goji berry)

4 cups hot water

4 cups cold water

1. In a large glass container like an 8-cup measuring cup, place the Ju hua, Da zao, and Gou qi zi, and add the hot water.

2. Infuse, covering if possible, for at least 15 minutes. If you are adding other teas, include them in the infusion.

3. Once the herbs have infused, strain out the herbs and add the cold water. Enjoy liberally.

Hot and Humid Summer Cooler

MAKES 8 CUPS

The heat and humidity of summer (especially as the season wears on) can build up and leave you feeling tired, lethargic, and uncomfortable. Ju hua (chrysanthemum) paired with Yi yi ren (Job's tears) cools and helps drain that summer Dampness. Hibiscus is a cooling summer favorite that pairs well with Ju hua.

¼ cup Ju hua (chrysanthemum)

1 tablespoon Yi yi ren (Job's tears)

4 cups hot water

4 cups cold water

1. In a large glass container like an 8-cup measuring cup, place the Ju hua and Yi yi ren and add the hot water.

2. Infuse, covering if possible, for at least 15 minutes. If you are adding other teas, include them in the infusion.

3. Once the herbs have infused, strain out the herbs and add the cold water. Enjoy throughout the day.

Vision

Healthy vision is supported by the Liver and nourished by Blood. For chronic eye problems, addressing patterns like Blood deficiency is recommended. Allergies, colds, and environmental factors can also lead to Heat and irritation in the eyes.

Eye Soak for Red, Itchy Eyes

MAKES 1 SERVING OF TEA AND 2 TEA BAGS

Ju hua (chrysanthemum) is a premiere herb for the eyes, clearing Heat to relieve redness, itchiness, and dryness.

2 to 3 tablespoons Ju hua (chrysanthemum)

2 empty tea bags

Water

1. Over a plate or towel, fill the tea bags with the Ju hua.
2. Place the tea bags in a large mug and pour boiling water over them.
3. Cover the mixture and infuse for 15 minutes.
4. Squeeze excess liquid out of the tea bags, remove, and place in a bowl.
5. Drink the infusion while the tea bags cool. Once they are cool, sit back and relax with a tea bag over each eye.

Infusion for Irritated Eyes

MAKES 1 CUP

This infusion uses Ju hua (chrysanthemum) to cool and soothe red, irritated eyes. Bo he (mint) works with Ju hua to cool while helping resolve colds or allergies.

1 tablespoon Ju hua (chrysanthemum)

1 teaspoon Bo he (mint)

Water

1. Place the Ju hua and Bo he in a large mug.
2. Pour boiling water over the herbs, cover, and infuse for 15 minutes.
3. Strain and drink. Repeat up to 3 times per day.

Decoction for Floaters in the Vision

MAKES 7 CUPS

Floaters in the visual field are due to the pattern of Liver Blood deficiency. Any formula that builds Liver Blood or Yin can help, but here Gou qi zi (goji berry) and Ju hua (chrysanthemum) are the archetypal pair for eye health. To support the health of your eyes and vision, Gou qi zi helps nourish Liver Blood, and Ju hua helps clear any Heat. It takes time to build Yin, so use this formula consistently to see results. Bai shao (peony) further builds Liver Blood to assist Gou qi zi.

21 grams Gou qi zi
   (goji berry)

21 grams Bai shao (peony)

8 cups water

12 grams Ju hua
   (chrysanthemum)

1. Place the Gou qi zi and Bai shao in a non-aluminum stockpot and add the water.

2. Bring the mixture to a boil, then simmer uncovered for 30 minutes.

3. Add the Ju hua and simmer for another 5 minutes.

4. Strain into a large, 8-cup glass measuring cup. If the total amount is less than 7 cups, add water to bring it to 7 cups total.

5. Set aside ½ cup as the first dose to drink immediately, then refrigerate the rest.

6. Drink ½ cup morning and evening for 1 week. After 7 days, discard any remaining decoction and make a new batch.

Weight-Loss Support

TCM patterns of disharmony show that there is no one right answer for weight loss. Those trying to lose weight can become frustrated that they work hard without the results they desire. There is a reason the weight-loss industry is as large as it is! Chinese herbal medicine can help by treating any patterns of disharmony and bringing balance to support weight-loss efforts.

First, making sure the Spleen Qi is strong and able to do its job and that digestion overall is optimal can significantly support weight loss by supplying energy and helping your body access adequate nutrients. When your Earth element is replete and balanced, you have more energy to put into caring for yourself.

Second, TCM sees excess weight as Dampness, although I find this overly simplistic and never an answer by itself. Draining Dampness helps tonify the Spleen, and if you truly have excess and mismanaged fluids, it can clear up imbalances that impede weight loss. While it can help, it is only one piece of the puzzle.

Third, helping balance emotions and stress can be a huge help if stresses get in the way of self-care or if emotional eating is an issue. Clearing any Qi stagnation causing stuck emotions, or soothing anxiety and frustration, can be very beneficial. Meditation and having a calm, mindful center from which to live life can positively impact weight loss.

Fourth, getting deep, truly restful sleep improves all areas of your health. Supplementing Blood and Yin to help with deep sleep and clearing any stagnation or Heat that may be in the way will help build energy and balance, helping with weight loss.

Finally, you need to balance any remaining conditions and temperature. For example, cold conditions slow things down, and if someone is Yang deficient and cold, it can lead to slower digestion and metabolism and inertia when it comes to moving and exercising to support weight loss. The other side is that Heat and Yin deficiency also cause problems—for example, Stomach Heat causing excess hunger.

At least one formula for each of these five areas is included in this section.

Decoction to Support Weight Loss and Spleen Qi

MAKES 7 CUPS

Spleen Qi is in charge of your energy: the energy to absorb nutrients from your food, the energy to get work done, and the energy to take care of yourself. When you need energy, you may look for it in quick, convenient foods like sugar and caffeine. This formula can give you extra energy and help keep your blood sugar balanced. It can also give you energy to form new, healthier lifestyle habits.

21 grams Bai zhu (atractylodes)

12 grams Huang qi (astragalus)

9 grams Fu ling (poria)

9 grams Da zao (dates)

8 cups water

1. Place the Bai zhu, Huang qi, Fu ling, and Da zao in a non-aluminum stockpot and add the water.

2. Bring the mixture to a boil, then simmer uncovered for 25 minutes. Remove from the heat.

3. Strain into a large, 8-cup glass measuring cup. If the total amount is less than 7 cups, add water to bring it to 7 cups total.

4. Set aside ½ cup as the first dose to drink immediately, then refrigerate the rest.

5. Drink ½ cup morning and evening for 1 week. After 7 days, discard any remaining decoction and make a new batch.

Decoction to Support Weight Loss and Drain Dampness

MAKES 7 CUPS

If there is excess Dampness, these two herbs can be decocted alone or, preferably, added to the Decoction to Support Weight Loss and Spleen Qi (page 178).

12 grams Yi yi ren (Job's tears)

12 grams Chen pi (tangerine peel)

8 cups water

1. Place the Yi yi ren and Chen pi in a non-aluminum stockpot and add the water.

2. Bring the mixture to a boil, then simmer uncovered for 25 minutes. Remove from the heat.

3. Strain into a large, 8-cup glass measuring cup. If the total amount is less than 7 cups, add water to bring it to 7 cups total.

4. Set aside ½ cup as the first dose to drink immediately, then refrigerate the rest.

5. Drink ½ cup morning and evening for 1 week. After 7 days, discard any remaining decoction and make a new batch.

PRECAUTIONS: Do not use if there is dryness or Heat.

Fenugreek for Weight-Loss Support

MAKES 1 CUP

Hu lu ba (fenugreek) has significant research backing up its work supporting maintaining a healthy weight, cholesterol, and blood sugar. Whole seeds can be hard to find in grocery stores, but they are available online or at your local Indian grocer (called *methi* in Hindi). One French study in the *European Journal of Clinical Pharmacology* found that patients taking Hu lu ba consumed less fat and fewer calories, supporting long-term weight loss. Fenugreek seeds are very hard and have to be cooked before eating. While simply soaking overnight creates a fenugreek infusion, I prefer the decoction method, which further softens the Hu lu ba seeds so that their helpful fiber can be consumed along with the decoction.

1 tablespoon Hu lu ba (fenugreek), whole seeds

1 cup water

SOAKING METHOD:

1. Place the whole Hu lu ba seeds in a bowl or glass jar and add the water.

2. Soak overnight.

3. Strain and drink before one or all meals. To make a larger batch, increase to 5 tablespoons Hu lu ba and 5 cups water. Refrigerate the excess and drink within 3 days.

DECOCTION METHOD:

1. Place the whole Hu lu ba seeds in a non-aluminum saucepan and add the water.

2. Bring the mixture to a boil, and simmer for 10 minutes. Remove from the heat.

3. Continue soaking the Hu lu ba mixture for a few hours or overnight.

4. Drink the decoction. You can drink the soaked seeds, eat them, or add them to dishes.

5. To make a larger batch, increase to 5 tablespoons Hu lu ba and 5 cups water. Refrigerate the excess and drink within 3 days.

Decoction to Support Weight Loss and Reduce Stress

MAKES 7 CUPS

This formula helps calm emotions to ease stress. Stress can raise cortisol levels, which can make losing weight more difficult and can also lead to emotional eating.

15 grams Gou qi zi (goji berry)

12 grams Long yan rou (longan)

12 grams He huan pi (albizzia peel)

8 cups water

1. Place the Gou qi zi, Long yan rou, and He huan pi in a non-aluminum cooking pot and add the water.

2. Bring the mixture to a boil, then simmer uncovered for 25 minutes. Remove from the heat.

3. Strain into a large, 8-cup glass measuring cup. If the total amount is less than 7 cups, add water to bring it to 7 cups total.

4. Set aside ½ cup as the first dose to drink immediately, then refrigerate the rest.

5. Drink ½ cup morning and evening for 1 week. After 7 days, discard any remaining decoction and make a new batch.

Infusion to Support Weight Loss and Calm Emotions

MAKES UP TO 4 CUPS

The Decoction to Support Weight Loss and Reduce Stress (page 181) is meant to be taken twice a day, but this Calm Emotions infusion can be taken anytime during the day to help with nerves, anxiety, uneasy feelings, palpitations, or tightness in the chest. Stress can raise cortisol levels, which can make losing weight more difficult and can also lead to emotional eating. If you carry a water bottle, you can keep infused Mei gui hua (rosebud) to drink throughout the day.

¼ cup Mei gui hua
    (rosebud)

Boiling water

Tea bags (optional for
    take-to-work method)

OVERNIGHT INFUSING METHOD:

1. Before bed, place the Mei gui hua in a teapot and add the boiling water.

2. Infuse overnight. Strain the mixture.

3. Drink the infusion throughout the next day, either warm or cool, diluting to your preferred taste.

TAKE-TO-WORK METHOD:

1. Fill the tea bags with the Mei gui hua (the number of tea bags will depend on the size of tea bags purchased).

2. Put the tea bags in a storage container and use them throughout the day, wherever you are.

3. To prepare the tea, place 1 tea bag in a mug and add hot water, covering and allowing it to infuse for up to 15 minutes.

Decoction to Support Weight Loss and Manage Stress

MAKES UP TO 4 CUPS

He huan hua (albizzia flower) has a different energetic than Mei gui hua (rosebud). Mei gui hua can be cooling and moving, where He huan hua is calming but a little less moving than Mei gui hua. Instead of the coolness of Mei gui hua, He huan hua has a neutral temperature while soothing nerves, anxiety, uneasy feelings, palpitations, or tightness in the chest.

¼ cup **He huan hua** (albizzia flower)

Boiling water

Tea bags (optional for take-to-work method)

OVERNIGHT INFUSING METHOD:

1. Before bed, place the He huan hua in a teapot and add the boiling water.
2. Infuse overnight. Strain the mixture.
3. Drink the infusion throughout the next day, either warm or cool, diluting to your preferred taste.

TAKE-TO-WORK METHOD:

1. Fill the tea bags with the He huan hua (the number of tea bags will depend on the size of tea bags purchased).
2. Put the tea bags in a storage container and use them throughout the day, wherever you are.
3. To prepare the tea, place 1 tea bag in a mug and add hot water, covering and allowing it to infuse for up to 15 minutes.

Infusion to Support Weight Loss and Calm a Nervous Stomach

MAKES UP TO 4 CUPS

Emotions such as anxiety and nervousness aren't always felt in the chest; sometimes they manifest as mild nausea or upset in the stomach, like the feeling described by the phrase *butterflies in the stomach*. Da zao (dates) nourishes the Stomach and Spleen, calming them, while Chen pi (tangerine peel) settles nausea, adding warmth to the Stomach and Spleen.

4 to 6 pieces Da zao (dates)

2 tablespoons Chen pi
   (tangerine peel)

Boiling water

1. Before bed, place the Da zao and Chen pi in a teapot and add the boiling water. Infuse overnight.

2. Drink throughout the day, either warm or cool.

Decoction to Support Weight Loss and Quality Sleep

MAKES 7 CUPS

Truly restful sleep improves all areas of health and is an important component of maintaining a healthy weight. This formula is best taken in the evening an hour before bed.

18 grams He huan pi (albizzia peel)

12 grams Bai shao (peony)

9 grams Tian men dong (asparagus root)

9 grams Da zao (dates)

6 grams Dan shen (salvia)

8 cups water

1. Place the He huan pi, Bai shao, Tian men dong, Da zao, and Dan shen in a non-aluminum stockpot and add the water.

2. Bring the mixture to a boil, then simmer uncovered for 25 minutes. Remove from the heat.

3. Strain into a large, 8-cup glass measuring cup. If the total amount is less than 7 cups, add water to bring it to 7 cups total.

4. Set aside ½ cup as the first dose to drink immediately, then refrigerate the rest.

5. Drink ½ cup morning and evening for 1 week. After 7 days, discard any remaining decoction and make a new batch.

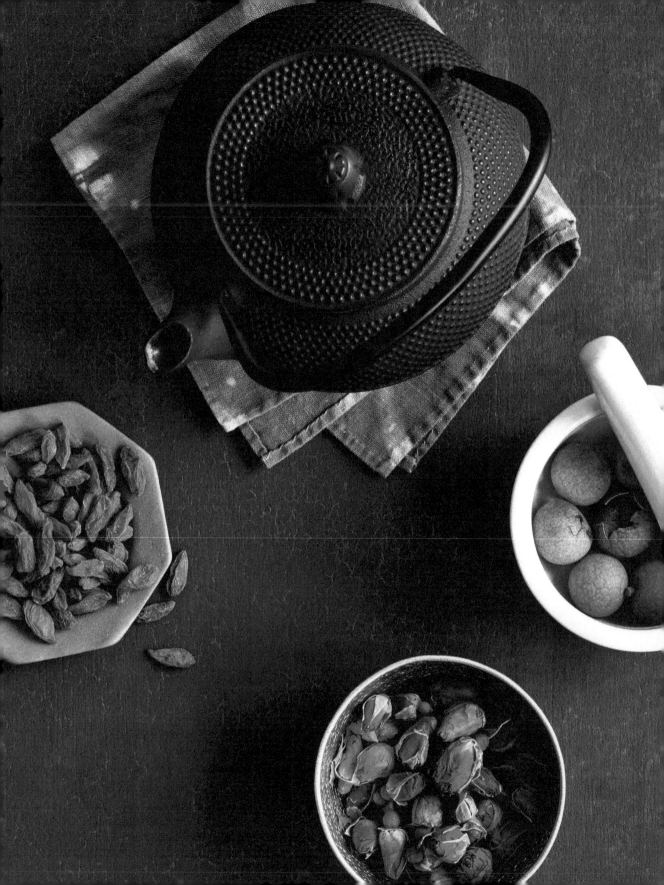

Resources

TO PURCHASE HERBS OR SEEDS

Five Flavors Herbs: FiveFlavorsHerbs.com

Jean's Greens: JeansGreens.com

Lilium Initiative (for sustainable, increased growing of Asian herbs in the United States): Liliuminitiative.org

Mountain Rose Herbs: MountainRoseHerbs.com

Strictly Medicinal Seeds: StrictlyMedicinalSeeds.com

Spring Wind Herbs: SpringWind.com

TO PURCHASE TOPICALS

There are many companies producing topicals, but these three are companies that offer quality products following GMP standards.

Plum Dragon. Focused on martial arts formulas, this company's products can be used for all sorts of pain and injuries from any cause. Plum Dragon gets one thing right that so many don't: their packaging. I have rings from oils and liniments where using the bottle causes a mess. This company uses a classic brown glass bottle with dropper, and the dropper means their products are the easiest to use and the least messy. PlumDragonHerbs.com

Blue Poppy is a trusted manufacturer of Chinese herbal products. They are also a leader in education and publishing for TCM practitioners. BluePoppy.com

Kamwo produces a line of topicals in conjunction with Tom Bisio called Tooth from the Tiger's Mouth. These formulas are clearly divided for use according to the stage of the injury, from acute to chronic. KamwoHerbs.com

References

Aggarwal, Bharat B. *Healing Spices: How to Use 50 Everyday and Exotic Spices to Boost Health and Beat Disease*. With Debora Yost. New York: Sterling, 2011.

Bai, Ye, Kun Li, Jiayao Shao, Qiuxiang Luo, and Li Hua Jin. "*Flos Chrysanthemi indici* Extract Improves a High-Sucrose Diet-Induced Metabolic Disorder in *Drosophila*." *Experimental and Therapeutic Medicine* 16, no. 3 (September 2018): 2564–72. https://doi.org/10.3892/etm.2018.6470.

Bensky, Dan, Steven Clavey, and Erich Stöger. *Chinese Herbal Medicine: Materia Medica*. 3rd edition. With Andrew Gamble. Illustrations adapted by Lilian Lai Bensky. Seattle: Eastland Press, 2004.

Bisio, Tom. *A Tooth from the Tiger's Mouth: How to Treat Your Injuries with Powerful Healing Secrets of the Great Chinese Warriors*. New York: Fireside, 2004.

Block, Jason P., Yulei He, Alan M. Zaslavsky, Lin Ding, and John Z. Ayanian. "Psychosocial Stress and Change in Weight among US Adults." *American Journal of Epidemiology* 170, no. 2 (July 15, 2009): 181–92. https://doi.org/10.1093/aje/kwp104.

Blue Poppy. Accessed December 30, 2019. http://www.BluePoppy.com.

Brusselaers, Nele, Karl Wahlin, Lars Engstrand, and Jesper Lagergren. "Maintenance Therapy with Proton Pump Inhibitors and Risk of Gastric Cancer: A Nationwide Population-Based Cohort Study in Sweden." *BMJ Open* 7, no. 10 (October 30, 2017). https://doi.org/10.1136/bmjopen-2017-017739.

Caldecott, Todd. *Food as Medicine: The Theory and Practice of Food*. Vancouver, BC: PhytoAlchemy, 2011.

Caldecott, Todd. *Inside Ayurveda: Clinical Education for the Western Practitioner*. Vancouver, BC: PhytoAlchemy, 2013.

Chen, Li-Chun, Bo-Kai Jiang, Wen-Hao Zheng, Shi-Yu Zhang, Jia-Jiang Li, and Zhong-Yang Fan. "Preparation, Characterization and Anti-diabetic Activity of Polysaccharides from Adlay Seed." *International Journal of Biological Macromolecules* 139 (October 15, 2019): 605–13. https://doi.org/10.1016/j.ijbiomac.2019.08.018.

Chevassus, Hugues, Jean-Baptiste Gaillard, Anne Farret, Françoise Costa, Isabelle Gabillaud, Emilie Mas, Anne-Marie Dupuy, et al. "A Fenugreek Seed Extract Selectively Reduces Spontaneous Fat Intake in Overweight Subjects." *European Journal of Clinical Pharmacology* 66, no. 5 (May 2010): 449–55. https://doi.org/10.1007/s00228-009-0770-0.

Daubenmier, Jennifer, Jean Kristeller, Frederick M. Hecht, Nicole Maninger, Margaret Kuwata, Kinnari Jhaveri, Robert H. Lustig, Margaret Kemeny, Lori Karan, and Elissa Epel. "Mindfulness Intervention for Stress Eating to Reduce Cortisol and Abdominal Fat among Overweight and Obese Women: An Exploratory Randomized Controlled Study." *Journal of Obesity* (2011). https://doi.org/10.1155/2011/651936.

Garran, Thomas Avery. *Western Herbs According to Traditional Chinese Medicine: A Practitioner's Guide*. Rochester, VT: Healing Arts Press, 2008.

Hsu, Ching Hsiang, Chun Mei Lu, and Tung Ti Chang. "Efficacy and Safety of Modified Mai-Men-Dong-Tang for Treatment of Allergic Asthma." *Pediatric Allergy and Immunology* 16, no. 1 (February 2005): 76–81. https://doi.org/10.1111/j.1399-3038.2005.00230.x.

Kamwo Meridian Herbs. "Tooth from the Tiger's Mouth." Accessed December 30, 2019. https://kamwoherbs.com/tooth-from.

Kang, Nu Ri, Bo-Jeong Pyun, Dong Ho Jung, Ik Soo Lee, Chan-Sik Kim, Young Sook Kim, and Jin Sook Kim. "*Pueraria lobata* Extract Protects Hydrogen Peroxide-Induced Human Retinal Pigment Epithelial Cells Death and Membrane Permeability." *Evidence-Based Complementary and Alternative Medicine* (August 27, 2019). https://doi.org/10.1155/2019/5710289.

Lee, Do Yeon, Goya Choi, Taesook Yoon, Myeong Sook Cheon, Byung Kil Choo, and Ho Kyoung Kim. "Anti-inflammatory Activity of *Chrysanthemum indicum* Extract in Acute and Chronic Cutaneous Inflammation." *Journal of Ethnopharmacology* 123, no. 1 (May 4, 2009): 149–54. https://doi.org/10.1016/j.jep.2009.02.009.

Liu, Ping, Haiping Zhao, and Yumin Luo. "Anti-aging Implications of *Astragalus membranaceus* (Huangqi): A Well-Known Chinese Tonic." *Aging and Disease* 8, no. 6 (December 2017): 868–86. https://doi.org/10.14336/AD.2017.0816.

Nyklíček, Ivan, Paula M. C. Mommersteeg, Sylvia Van Beugen, Christian Ramakers, and Geert J. Van Boxtel. "Mindfulness-Based Stress Reduction and Physiological Activity during Acute Stress: A Randomized Controlled Trial." *Health Psychology* 32, no. 10 (October 2013): 1110–13. https://doi.org/10.1037/a0032200.

Penetar, David M., Lindsay H. Toto, David Y.-W. Lee, and Scott E. Lukas. "A Single Dose of Kudzu Extract Reduces Alcohol Consumption in a Binge Drinking Paradigm." *Drug and Alcohol Dependence* 153 (August 1, 2015): 194–200. https://doi.org/10.1016/j.drugalcdep.2015.05.025.

Plum Dragon. Accessed December 30, 2019. http://www.PlumDragonHerbs.com.

Strictly Medicinal Seeds. Accessed December 30, 2019. http://www.strictlymedicinalseeds.com.

Taylor, David A. "The Fight against Ginseng Poaching in the Great Smoky Mountains." *Smithsonian Magazine*. Last modified April 21, 2016. https://www.smithsonianmag.com/science-nature/fight-against-ginseng-poaching-great-smoky-mountains-180958858/.

Texas Invasive Species Institute. Accessed December 30, 2019. http://www.tsusinvasives.org.

USDA Natural Resource Conservation Service. "*Cyperus rotundus* L." Accessed December 30, 2019. https://plants.usda.gov/core/profile?symbol=CYRO.

Wachtel-Galor, Sissi, John Yuen, John A. Buswell, and Iris F. F. Benzie. "*Ganoderma lucidum* (Lingzhi or Reishi): A Medicinal Mushroom." In *Herbal Medicine: Biomolecular and Clinical Aspects*, edited by Iris F. F. Benzie and Sissi Wachtel-Galor. 2nd edition. Boca Raton, FL: CRC Press/Taylor & Francis, 2011.

Walker, Josh. *Materia Medica for Martial Artists*. CreateSpace Independent Publishing Platform, 2012.

Wang, Jue, Bin Cao, Haiping Zhao, and Juan Feng. "Emerging Roles of *Ganoderma lucidum* in Anti-aging." *Aging and Disease* 8, no. 6 (December 2017): 691–707. https://doi.org/10.14336/AD.2017.0410.

Wang, Li Ying, Kam Wa Chan, Ya Yuwen, Nan Nan Shi, Xue Jie Han, and Aiping Lu. "Expert Consensus on the Treatment of Hypertension with Chinese Patent Medicines." *Evidence-Based Complementary and Alternative Medicine* (2013). https://doi.org/10.1155/2013/510146.

Wang, Liwen, Jinhan Wang, Lianying Fang, Zuliang Zheng, Dexian Zhi, Suying Wang, Shiming Li, Chi-Tang Ho, and Hui Zhao. "Anticancer Activities of Citrus Peel Polymethoxyflavones Related to Angiogenesis and Others." *BioMed Research International* (August 28, 2014). https://doi.org/10.1155 /2014 /453972.

Yang, Pei-Rung, Wei-Tai Shih, Yen-Hua Chu, Pau-Chung Chen, and Ching-Yuan Wu. "Frequency and Co-prescription Pattern of Chinese Herbal Products for Hypertension in Taiwan: A Cohort Study." *BMC Complementary and Alternative Medicine* 15 (2015): 163. https://doi.org/10.1186/s12906-015-0690-8.

Yu, Ping, Si Cheng, Juan Xiang, Bin Yu, Mian Zhang, Chaofeng Zhang, and Xianghong Xu. "Expectorant, Antitussive, Anti-inflammatory Activities and Compositional Analysis of *Aster tataricus.*" *Journal of Ethnopharmacology* 164 (April 22, 2015): 328–33. https://doi.org/10.1016/j.jep.2015.02.036.

Zhang, Hongxia, Zheng Feei Ma, Xiaoqin Luo, and Xinli Li. "Effects of Mulberry Fruit (*Morus alba* L.) Consumption on Health Outcomes: A Mini-Review." *Antioxidants* (Basel) 7, no. 5 (May 2018): 69. https://doi.org/10.3390/antiox7050069.

Index

Acknowledgments

I AM GRATEFUL to Anuj, Akshay, and the rest of my family for their support. To Carrie Hura for being my inspirational sounding board and Cindy Lasley for encouragement. To the many teachers who have helped me move forward on this path. Thank you to the Academy for Five Element Acupuncture, especially Misti Oxford-Pickeral, Teresa Bruggeman, and Jim Brooks. The Herbal Dispensary at AFEA always felt like home. To Scott Blossom and Integrative Yoga Therapy for showing me how to empower individuals to care for themselves. To Thomas Avery Garran for forging a path for Chinese herbalists to use local herbs; to Todd Caldecott of the Dogwood School of Botanical Medicine. To the American Herbalists Guild and herbalists like Amanda McQuade Crawford for leading the way. Thanks to my editor Samantha Barbaro and Callisto Media for giving me the opportunity to write about something I absolutely love.

About the Author

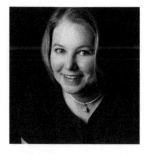

CARRIE CHAUHAN, MAc, DiplOM, has a master's in acupuncture and a Diplomate of Oriental Medicine. She practices Chinese herbal medicine flavored by her experience in Ayurveda, integrative yoga therapy, and Western herbal medicine. The former director of herbal studies at the Academy for Five Element Acupuncture in Florida, she is also a registered herbalist with the American Herbalists Guild. Carrie currently lives in Colorado, where she practices and writes while furthering her studies in herbal medicine, tae kwon do, and qigong. Find out more at CarrieChauhan.com.

Printed in the USA
CPSIA information can be obtained
at www.ICGtesting.com
LVHW071505041123
762724LV00002B/13